THE AUTOIMMUNE PROTOCOL
COMFORT
FOOD
COOKBOOK

100+ Nourishing Allergen-Free Recipes

Michelle Hoover, NTP
of *Unbound Wellness*

Foreword by Dr. Sarah Ballantyne, Ph.D.,
New York Times best-selling author of *The Paleo Approach*

FAIR WINDS

DEDICATION

This cookbook is dedicated with love to my amazing husband, Daniel, and, of course, to all the incredible readers of UnboundWellness.com.

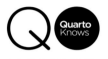

Brimming with creative inspiration, how-to projects, and useful information to enrich your everyday life, Quarto Knows is a favorite destination for those pursuing their interests and passions. Visit our site and dig deeper with our books into your area of interest: Quarto Creates, Quarto Cooks, Quarto Homes, Quarto Lives, Quarto Drives, Quarto Explores, Quarto Gifts, or Quarto Kids.

First Published in 2019 by Fair Winds Press, an imprint of The Quarto Group, 100 Cummings Center, Suite 265-D, Beverly, MA 01915, USA.
T (978) 282-9590 F (978) 283-2742 QuartoKnows.com

Fair Winds Press titles are also available at discount for retail, wholesale, promotional, and bulk purchase. For details, contact the Special Sales Manager by email at specialsales@quarto.com or by mail at The Quarto Group, Attn: Special Sales Manager, 100 Cummings Center, Suite 265-D, Beverly, MA 01915, USA.

23 22 21 20 19   1 2 3 4 5

ISBN: 978-1-59233-893-1

Digital edition published in 2019
eISBN: 978-1-59233-894-8

Library of Congress Cataloging-in-Publication Data available

Design: Samantha J. Bednarek
Cover Image: Michelle Hoover
Page Layout: Samantha J. Bednarek
Food Photography: Michelle Hoover
Chapter Opener Photography: Melanie Shafranek and Michelle Hoover
Headshot Photographer: Maribel Morales

Printed in China

The information in this book is for educational purposes only. It is not intended to replace the advice of a physician or medical practitioner. Please see your health-care provider before beginning any new health program.

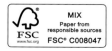

FOREWORD

DR. SARAH BALLANTYNE, PHD,
New York Times best-selling author of *The Paleo Approach*.

AUTOIMMUNE DISEASE IS EPIDEMIC in our society, as tens of millions deal with diagnoses ranging from multiple sclerosis, to Hashimoto's thyroiditis, to rheumatoid arthritis, to psoriasis, to lupus, and more—there are over 140 chronic diseases confirmed or suspected of falling under the autoimmune umbrella. The symptoms of autoimmune disease can have a severe impact on our daily lives, and overall vitality.

The Autoimmune Protocol, or AIP, is a template created for those struggling with autoimmune disease to reduce inflammation and support the body's natural ability to heal. Through its focus on selecting nutrient-dense, healing foods; eliminating inflammatory foods; and making specific lifestyle choices, quality of life can be drastically improved.

There is scientific evidence that the AIP is indeed effective. In a 2017 clinical trial of patients with Inflammatory Bowel Disease, 73 percent of participants experienced full remission within six weeks of starting the protocol. Similarly impressive results were seen in a 2019 clinical trial of Hashimoto's thyroiditis patients, who experienced a significant decrease in symptoms as measured by health-related quality of life scores, accompanied by lower markers of systemic inflammation, within the ten-week study period.

Though the AIP diet temporarily eliminates many foods that we are accustomed to enjoying in the context of holidays, celebrations, and other fun settings, there is still plenty of opportunity for enjoying comfort food made from nourishing and compliant ingredients! *The Autoimmune Protocol Comfort Food Cookbook* is a fantastic resource for those looking to enjoy nostalgic dishes, holiday classics, decadent treats, tasty snacks, and family favorites, all while on the AIP diet! This cookbook features over 100 creative and delicious recipes, written by Michelle Hoover, NTP, who has shared her popular AIP creations for several years on her blog.

Healthy living relies heavily on the foods that we eat and the choices that we make daily, but it is also dependent on the sense of community and human connection that we have in our lives. For thousands of years, humans have gathered around a common table to share, bond, and celebrate with food. *The Autoimmune Protocol Comfort Food Cookbook* allows you to share cherished comfort food flavors with loved ones while unreservedly enjoying nourishing AIP foods yourself!

Michelle aims to make sure that those who are following an Autoimmune Protocol diet—or who have food intolerances to gluten, dairy, soy, nightshade, nuts and more—are able to feel a sense of joy and abundance with the food that they eat. This book is your key to do just that!

CONTENTS

INTRODUCTION
My Autoimmune Healing Story
9

Loaded Baked Potato Soup, page 67 →

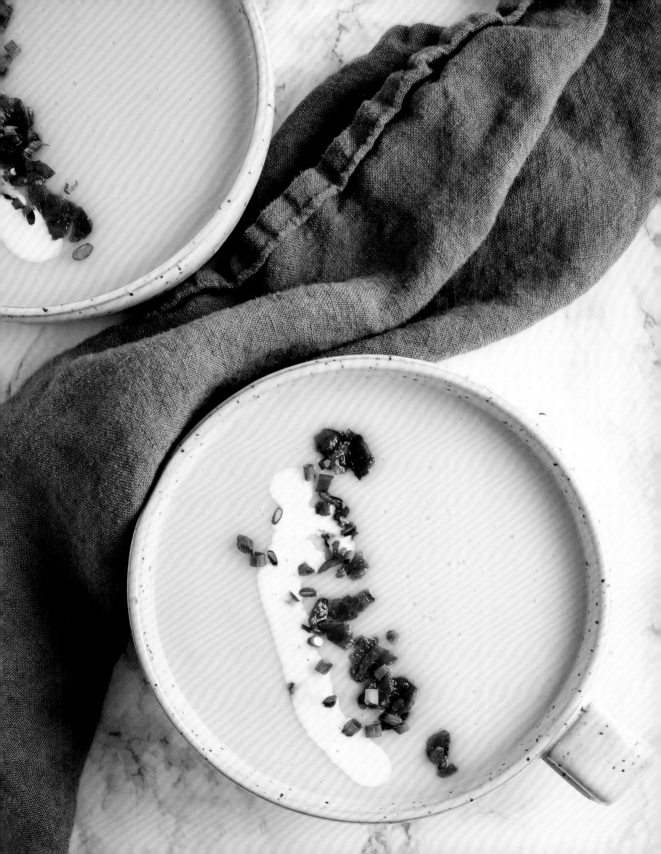

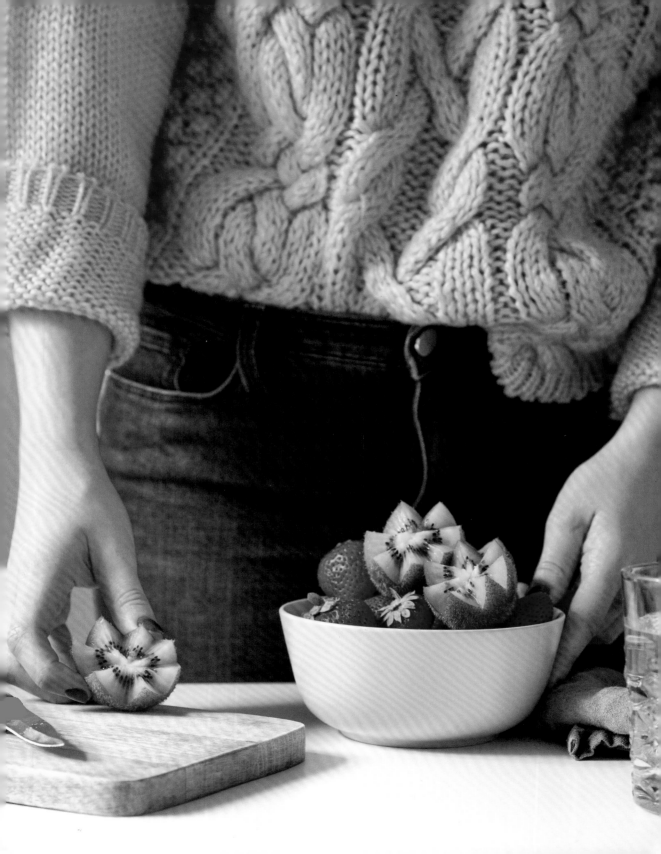

MY AUTOIMMUNE HEALING STORY

GROWING UP, I was never a healthy kid. I often experienced dizziness and usually had some kind of infection or stomachache. Although I was labeled a hypochondriac, everything changed at the age of 17 when I was diagnosed with Hashimoto's disease.

Hashimoto's is a disease in which the immune system attacks the thyroid gland, which is responsible for many of the body's functions. It is the most common cause of hypothyroidism, or underactive thyroid. Hashimoto's is a chronic condition. Signs include fatigue, depression, sensitivity to cold, joint aches, constipation, a puffy face, pale, dry skin, brittle nails, and more.

The diagnosis turned my life upside down. I was overwhelmed, confused, and scared for what the rest of my life would look like and plagued by myriad symptoms. I would sleep up to 18 hours a day, and I suffered from fainting spells, food intolerances, mood swings, weight changes, and more. Youth is supposed to be a vibrant, carefree time, but I felt like my body was deteriorating, my life was out of control, and that I was completely alone. Conventional medicine told me there was little I could do and certainly nothing I could do holistically. Though I was prescribed medication, it wasn't the right balance for my body and little changed.

After several years of battling debilitating symptoms, I learned about the gut connection to autoimmune disease, as well as possibly restoring my health with personalized functional, or alternative, medicine, different medication prescribed by my doctor, and real food—via the Autoimmune Protocol (AIP) diet. My doctor explained that our gut health is tied to our body's overall health, and when our gut health is compromised, it can trigger autoimmunity. After testing, I learned my gut health was severely compromised and several other aspects of my health needed support and rebalancing, including vitamin deficiencies, mineral imbalances, hormone imbalance, adrenal fatigue, and more. With personalized recommendations, such as proper supplementation, a new medication, and lifestyle changes such as healthy movement, I started to see they were having a positive effect on my life.

It took years for me to commit to a healing lifestyle. I often told myself that one little bite of pizza wouldn't hurt, or I would just start the diet on Monday. To me, giving up my favorite foods was unbearable. After weekly pity parties, I wound up back at the local gas station, buying and digging into bags of my favorite candy. Needless to say, I wasn't getting better. Things finally changed when I had one too many health scares and decided I needed to get serious. I finally shifted my mind-set away from obsessing over what I *couldn't* have to embracing what I *could* have. I stopped pining for grocery store cookies from a box and started experimenting and making my own cookies with ingredients that agreed with my body. I stopped telling myself I was unfortunate for not being able to eat delivery pizza without feeling ill and started feeling grateful for the foods that were nourishing my body and for feeling better physically when I made healthier choices. There were plenty of missteps, and this process took years, but it changed everything for me.

I adopted a healing lifestyle and found ways to make it fun by re-creating healthier versions of my favorite childhood foods, such as chicken nuggets and chocolate chip cookies. And, I felt so much better! My thyroid antibodies stabilized, my symptoms subsided, and I was inspired to go back to school to become a nutritional therapy practitioner and share my story and recipes on my blog, Unbound Wellness.com.

Although my health has improved, my healing journey is far from over. Since I was diagnosed with Hashimoto's, I've also dealt with numerous gut issues, such as food intolerances, as well as mercury toxicity, estrogen dominance, and obsessive-compulsive disorder. My lifestyle, outlook, and diet have made me better equipped to deal with these health challenges.

Above all, I've maintained a heart of gratitude for all the amazing things God has put in my life. Even in the darkest times, this faith helped me on my healing journey far more than all the kale in the world!

HAVING FUN WITH HEALTHY FOOD

When I first started a healing diet, it felt like the polar opposite of fun. Truthfully, that's what took so long for me to really commit and what kept me sick years longer than I needed to be. How was I supposed to have *fun* with my food if I couldn't enjoy Christmas cookies, Sunday-morning waffles, or hearty chili on a cool fall day? There had to be more than *just* kale and chicken for *every single meal*—right?

I took a step back and thought about the foods I used to love (and, as a major foodie, there were *a lot* of foods I loved) and wondered what I could do to adapt these foods to be allergen free and AIP friendly. After much trial and error in the kitchen, my diet slowly began to fill back up with the fun and comforting foods I love! Only I found I didn't *need* cane sugar, white flour, or shredded cheese—healthy ingredients, such as healthy fats, proteins, vegetables, and fruits, were all I needed! They're all you need, too, to prepare classic foods the whole family will love.

That's why this cookbook exists! I created the recipes here to help you eat the foods you love again, but without any inflammatory ingredients that stall healing. Comfort food can feature nutrient-dense ingredients and be delicious at the same time. These recipes allow you to enjoy old favorites on a healing diet and simply have fun planning a game day bash with Plantain Chips (page 59) and Queso Blanco (page 60), a birthday party with Chocolate Birthday Cupcakes with Pomegranate Frosting (page 180), a holiday dinner with Roasted Parsnip Mash (page 163), breakfast in bed with Blueberry Waffles (or Chicken and Waffle Sandwiches, if that's you thing!), or a cozy dinner in with Tuna Zoodle Casserole (page 152).

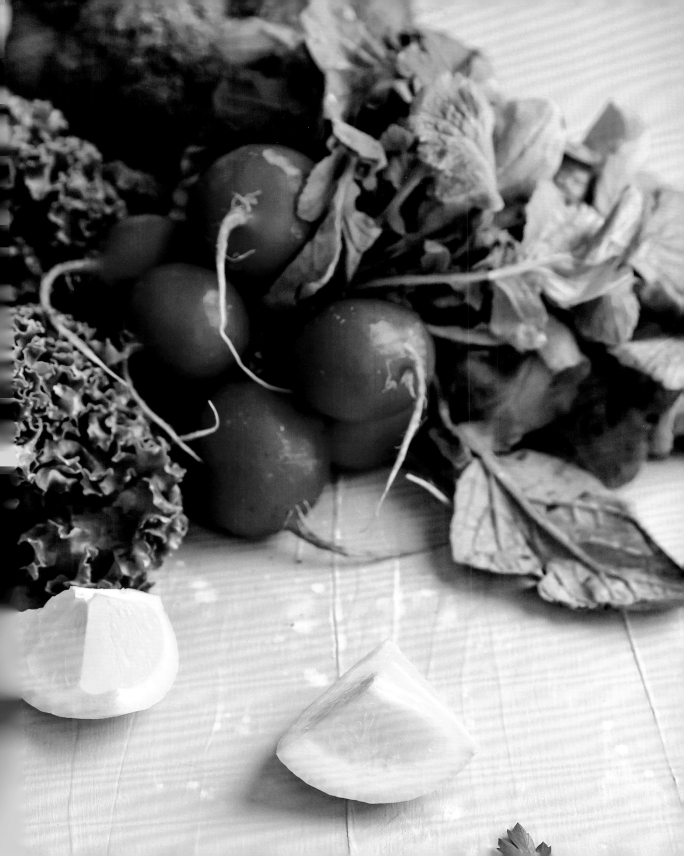

CHAPTER 1

ABOUT THE AUTOIMMUNE PROTOCOL

When first diagnosed with Hashimoto's disease as a teenager, diet was the furthest thing from my mind. I thought my symptoms were a life sentence and there was little I could do about it. It was only when I discovered the world of healing with food, through a gluten-free diet, then a paleo diet, and finally the autoimmune protocol, that I saw vast improvements to my health. If you suffer from any autoimmune disease, not just Hashimoto's, you may find success with this protocol. The AIP is designed to lower inflammation, in general, to allow the body to heal and rebalance.

In short, autoimmunity is characterized by the body attacking itself as if it were a foreign invader. This presents in a variety of ways depending on the particular autoimmunity disease. Inflammatory foods exacerbate the inflammation our body is already experiencing and can slow healing by adding more fuel to the fire.

Diet is not the only piece of the puzzle with autoimmunity and chronic illness, but it plays a large role, as it does with health in general. The AIP and holistic health community opened my eyes to a new way of living—starting with the new diet, focusing on better sleep, lowering my stress levels, and more positive healthy lifestyle changes—and helped me greatly improve and maintain my health. So, how do you get started? How do you still live a life of abundance after giving up some of your favorite foods?

AUTOIMMUNITY ON THE RISE

The National Institutes of Health (NIH) estimates up to 23.5 million Americans suffer from autoimmune disease and that the prevalence is rising. However, the American Autoimmune Related Diseases Association (AARDA) says that number is closer to 50 million, as the NIH only includes twenty-four diseases (of the many autoimmune diseases) with good epidemiology studies available.

As we've learned, autoimmunity is characterized by the body attacking itself as if it were a foreign invader. This is seen in Hashimoto's, as the immune system attacks the thyroid, in rheumatoid arthritis as the joints are under fire, and so on.

Nonetheless, no one person's autoimmunity is the same and various risk factors are involved. Some of the most common are as follows:

- Genetic predisposition
- Intestinal permeability (characterized by the tight junctions in the gut lining becoming damaged, allowing potentially harmful substances into the rest of the body and eliciting an overactive immune response and damage to the immune system within the gut)
- Physical or emotional stressors (e.g., stressful life events, infections, etc.)

Though there is no *cure* for autoimmunity and experiencing relief from symptoms doesn't happen overnight, symptoms may be effectively managed with a balance of Western and holistic interventions, such as the following:

- One-on-one care with a medical provider (e.g., functional medicine doctor, naturopath) and a customized protocol
- Addressing the underlying infections, nutritional imbalances, and so on
- Sleep and restorative lifestyle practices
- Customized exercise
- Community support
- Positive mind-set changes
- Spiritual practices
- Individualized healing diet

A CLOSER LOOK AT HEALING WITH FOOD

Healing with food alone? Is it really that simple? Yes and no. Yes, because food has a significant effect on our overall health and well-being, and the food we choose to consume can help repair and restore our health. No, because there's more to good health than food alone. There's also our mind-set, lifestyle, and more, which we'll get to later. First, we'll start with food.

What your grandma told you about food is true! We truly are what we eat. Healthy fats can reduce inflammation, lowering the risk for serious disease, such as cancer. The minerals in protein are essential for bone health, and the nutrients in vegetables lay the foundation for our overall health and vibrancy. If the majority of foods we consume are not health-promoting whole foods in their natural form, we can be putting our health at risk.

With every meal we eat, we have the opportunity to nourish our bodies with restorative foods to help us thrive. When we consider that, generally, we eat at least three times a day, every single day of our life, that's *a lot* of opportunity to make positive decisions for our health and well-being.

HOW THE AUTOIMMUNE PROTOCOL WORKS

The autoimmune protocol (AIP) is a diet template designed for those trying to heal autoimmunity, specifically to nourish the body with real, whole foods and eliminate inflammatory foods. A 2017 study published in *Inflammatory Bowel Diseases* (IBD) showed that the AIP improved symptoms of and reduced inflammation in patients with IBD during a six-week study followed by a five-week maintenance period. Thousands of people, including yours truly, rave about its efficacy in online communities!

The AIP diet is designed to be followed for a minimum of thirty days (though most follow it longer), along with positive lifestyle practices and working one on one with a health care practitioner.

After your symptoms subside to a noticeable degree, you slowly reintroduce foods—one at a time—and track your reactions. If a food reintroduction is successful, it is added back into your diet. If it fails, you keep the food out of your diet either long term or try another reintroduction attempt.

Why Does AIP Work?

While your autoimmune disease symptoms or issues are unique to you, overall, inflammatory foods are unhealthy for everyone—but especially those with an autoimmune disease who are dealing with excessive inflammation. So, this diet allows your immune system to take a break from dealing with inflammatory foods, such as grains, dairy, and nightshades, by removing them, which can potentially calm the inflammation. When the immune system calms down, we give our body the opportunity to heal. The nourishing foods on the autoimmune protocol give the body the proper vitamins, minerals, and nutrients to assist it in the healing process.

FOODS TO ENJOY

These health-promoting whole foods can be eaten daily.

VEGETABLES

Artichoke
Arugula
Asparagus
Beets
Bok choy
Broccoli
Brussels sprouts
Cabbage
Carrots
Cauliflower
Celery
Chard
Collards
Fennel
Garlic
Ginger
Jicama
Kale
Leeks
Lettuce
Mushrooms
Onions
Parsnips
Radishes
Rutabaga
Spinach
Squash
Sweet Potatoes
Yucca
Zucchini

HEALING SUPER FOODS

Foods such as bone broth and collagen powder are loaded with minerals and collagen that build a healthy gut and strong joints. Fermented foods have beneficial bacteria that influence a healthy immune system.

Beet kvass
Bone broth (beef, chicken, fish, lamb)
Collagen powder
Sauerkraut, and other fermented vegetables (you can ferment most any vegetable)
and foods such as water kefir or coconut kefir, coconut yogurt, etc.

PASTURED MEAT & WILD-CAUGHT FISH

Beef
Bison
Chicken
Crab
Duck
Lamb
Organ meats
Pork
Salmon
Sardines
Scallops
Shrimp
Trout
Tuna

HEALTHY FATS

Animal fats
Avocado
Coconut butter
Coconut oil
Olive oil
Palm oil

FRUIT

While refined sugar is a known inflammatory, natural sugar from fruit also comes with fiber and phytonutrients that aren't present in refined white sugars.

Apples
Bananas
Blackberries
Blueberries
Cranberries
Grapefruit
Lemons
Limes
Mangoes
Melon
Oranges
Peaches
Raspberries
Strawberries
Watermelon

HERBS & SPICES

Herbs and spices add extra nutrients and flavor to recipes, without unwanted sugar or salt.

Basil
Bay leaf
Chives
Cinnamon
Dill
Garlic
Ginger
Horseradish
Lavender
Parsley
Rosemary
Sage
Thyme
Turmeric

BAKING INGREDIENTS & SWEETENERS

Though these ingredients are to be to enjoyed **in moderation**, they come from whole food sources that are autoimmune protocol compliant and easier on the body than conventional refined desserts.

Arrowroot starch
Carob
Cassava flour
Coconut flour
Coconut sugar
Dates
Honey
Maple syrup/sugar
Molasses
Tapioca starch
Tigernut flour

FOODS TO AVOID

These foods can exacerbate inflammation and slow healing as a result. Though some may be reintroduced in the future, they are best eliminated for at least a thirty-day period during the protocol.

ALL GRAINS, GLUTEN, & PSEUDO GRAINS

Amaranth
Barley
Buckwheat
Bulger
Corn
Millet
Oats
Quinoa
Rice
Rye
Sorghum
Spelt
Wheat

DAIRY

Dairy is a very common intolerance, and the proteins in dairy can be damaging to the gut lining.

Butter
Cheese
Cream
Ghee
Milk
Yogurt

LEGUMES

Legumes contain *saponins*, which can be harmful to gut health.

Adzuki beans
Black beans
Black-eyed peas
Butter beans
Chickpeas
Green beans
Kidney beans
Lentils
Navy beans
Peanuts
Peas
Pinto beans
Red beans
Soy beans

EGGS

All eggs

NIGHTSHADES

The nightshade family includes tomatoes, potatoes, eggplant, all peppers, all red spices, and goji berries.

All peppers (sweet and hot)
Eggplant
Goji berries
Ground cherries
Paprika
Potatoes
Tomatillos
Tomatoes

NUTS & SEEDS

Almonds
Brazil nuts
Canola (rapeseed)
Cashews
Chestnuts
Chia seeds
Cocoa
Coffee
Hazelnuts
Hemp seeds
Pine nuts
Pistachios
Poppy seeds
Pumpkin seeds
Safflower
Sesame seeds
Walnuts

SEED-BASED SPICES

Black pepper
Clove
Coriander
Cumin
Fenugreek
Mustard seed
Nutmeg

REFINED SUGARS & ADDITIVES

Cane sugar
Carrageenan
Guar gum
Monosodium glutamate (MSG)
Nitrates/nitrites
Sulfates/sulfites
Xanthan gum

Finding Success with the Autoimmune Protocol

The list of foods to avoid can be a bit overwhelming, but don't panic! With the right action plan, you too can find success! Here's how:

• **Plan ahead.** When it comes to huge dietary changes, failing to plan is planning to fail. All it takes is a few minutes each week to sit down and map out what you plan to eat, make a shopping list, and make a plan to cook ahead of time. Taking time to meal prep some staple dishes each Sunday can save you hours in the kitchen throughout the week! It takes time to get into the habit of planning ahead, but it's worth the effort. This cookbook lists meal-prep ready meals you can serve throughout the week.

• **Work one-on-one with your health care provider.** It's crucial to have the support of a health care provider throughout your healing journey, whether a functional medicine doctor, naturopath, holistic chiropractor, or other professional. Food is a powerful tool, but it can only do so much. We need one-on-one customized medical attention to address deep-rooted infections, imbalances, and other health issues.

• **Track your symptoms and keep records of medical testing.** All too often, we don't notice the day-to-day changes unless we write them down! Keep a journal to track your major symptoms daily. You may be surprised with the changes you see, and your findings will help guide your progress.

• **Get community support.** Community support is one of the most essential foundations to a healthy lifestyle. The human race itself is meant to be in community, and finding your community can change everything. Whether it be online communities, in small church groups, or from strong family and friendship ties, human connection truly matters.

• **Remember, it's not all about the food.** You need to address other factors as well. Beyond working with a health care provider to address root causes, positive lifestyle changes such as getting enough exercise and sleep, reducing stress, and adjusting your mind-set are also crucial to long-term success!

• **Give yourself permission to have fun.** I know this process seems daunting. That thought is what held me back so long. However, it doesn't have to be. This protocol can be filled with an abundance of foods you love. Use this cookbook and other resources to keep things interesting while integrating the AIP into your life!

REINTRODUCING FOODS

The AIP is not meant to last forever. Rather, it gives your body time to heal and, potentially, tolerate certain foods in the future.

Though the process varies for everyone, many generally begin to reintroduce foods after following the AIP for at least thirty days and once you and your health care provider see a reduction in symptoms and improvement in your health. If a reintroduction is not successful and you experience a flare of symptoms, it may be a sign you still have more healing to do. However, some foods may not ever be fully reintroduced. You may experience one or more of the following symptoms after a reintroduction:

• **Digestive reactions**
• **Fatigue**
• **Headaches**
• **Hives, rashes, or flushing**
• **Joint pain**
• **Mood swings**
• **Sleep disturbances**

The Reintroduction Phases

In the reintroduction phases, foods are reintroduced in order of least inflammatory to most inflammatory. There is no standard for how long each phase lasts, and everyone takes the reintroduction process at their own pace. As you proceed with the reintroductions, each food you reintroduce successfully, with no associated symptoms, can be included then as a regular part of your diet. If you have a bad reaction and

THE FOUR PHASES

PHASE 1 FOODS
Coffee (occasional basis)
Cocoa and dark chocolate
Egg yolks
Grass-fed ghee
High-quality seed and nut oils
(sesame oil, almond oil, etc.)
Legumes (peas and green beans)
Seed-based spices

PHASE 2 FOODS
Alcohol (in small quantities)
Chia seeds
Coffee (daily basis)
Egg whites
Grass-fed butter
Nuts (almonds, Brazil nuts, hazelnuts,
macadamias, pecans, walnuts)
Seeds

PHASE 3 FOODS
Bell peppers
Eggplant
Fermented dairy
Grass-fed cream
Grass-fed whole milk
Paprika

PHASE 4 FOODS
Chile peppers
Nightshade spices, which include cayenne,
curry spice, and red pepper flakes
Potatoes
Soaked and sprouted grains
Soaked and sprouted legumes
Tomatoes
White rice

experience symptoms, the best course of action then is to lean back into healing foods such as bone broth, water, vegetable-rich meals, and fermented foods and give your body time to rest and recover before moving on to more reintroductions.

To effectively reintroduce potentially inflammatory foods back into your diet, follow this process:

1. Start with the Phase 1 foods (see sidebar).
2. Reintroduce one food at a time (do not reintroduce multiple new foods at once) and wait three days to gauge a reaction.
3. Track your reactions in your food journal. You're looking for responses such as headaches, mood swings, skin changes, fatigue, bloating, and so on.
4. Add foods that work to your regular rotation and restrict the foods that don't.
5. Repeat the process with the next food.

LIFE AFTER AIP
The AIP is designed to be a short-term healing protocol. However, life after the AIP should still incorporate the same healthy lifestyle principles of eating high-quality whole foods, working with a health care practitioner, practicing self-care, and so forth.

Many people who complete the diet and experience positive effects on their health still enjoy AIP recipes and AIP resets and remain in the AIP community for ongoing support for living well with autoimmunity. I still avoid the majority of grains as well as all nightshades and certain other foods and find amazing health benefits from a long-term diet based on an AIP template. Look to this cookbook not just for a 30-day protocol, but as a part of a healthy diet for life.

COOKBOOK INGREDIENTS GUIDE
Shopping for new and unfamiliar ingredients can be a challenge. This section gives you more insights into the ingredients used in the recipes.

Anchovies Use anchovies packed in olive oil or water and that do not contain any seed oils.

Arrowroot starch Also known as arrowroot flour, this starch is derived from a tropical root vegetable. Arrowroot is great for baking and can often be substituted with tapioca starch.

Artichoke hearts Artichoke hearts often are canned with citric acid. Look for canned artichokes without citric acid or frozen artichoke hearts.

Beef tallow Beef tallow is rendered beef fat and can be made at home or purchased at farmer's markets and health food stores.

Cassava flour Cassava flour is derived from the yucca plant and can be purchased online or in many stores.

Coconut aminos Use this as a substitute for soy sauce. Even gluten-free soy sauce is still soy based, which makes it noncompliant with the AIP. You can find this ingredient online and in most health food stores.

Coconut butter Also known as coconut cream concentrate or coconut mana, this is different from coconut oil. Coconut butter has a creamier texture and includes the meat of the coconut. This is sold in most grocery stores in the nut butter section.

Coconut cream You can purchase this in a can or make it yourself by placing full-fat coconut milk in the fridge overnight and using the hardened cream on top.

Coconut flour This is a common ingredient used in AIP baking that can't be easily substituted. The coconut-free recipes are labeled in this book, and I would not recommend swapping coconut flour for other flours as it doesn't swap one to one.

Coconut milk If you're buying premade coconut milk, watch out for gums and thickeners by reading the ingredients list.

Coconut sugar This unprocessed sugar is great in baked goods! You can find it in most stores.

Collagen Collagen is broken down gelatin derived from the bones, joints, and skin of animals. It adds a protein boost to recipes as well as gut and joint healing benefits.

Gelatin Gelatin is derived from the same source as collagen and can be used as an egg substitute in recipes such as Orange Turmeric Gummies (page 184).

Honey Try to find a local raw honey for the best quality product possible. If you prefer, substitute maple syrup in a 1:1 ratio.

Horseradish Horseradish is a great way to add spice without nightshades! You can buy horseradish powder online.

Maple syrup I love using maple syrup in baked goods! You can often swap honey at a ratio of 1:1.

Matcha powder Matcha is a green tea powder that yields a beautiful green color. You can save money by using culinary matcha if you're only using it for color, but it is also great as a cold or hot tea beverage.

Nutritional yeast Nutritional yeast lends a cheesy flavor in recipes such as Cauliflower "Mac & Cheese" (page 90). This can be found at health food stores and online.

Palm shortening Palm shortening is different than palm oil and gives body to recipes such as the frosting for the Gingerbread Cookies (page 167) or Mint Chip Brownies (page 179) and a cakey texture to baked goods. Coconut oil isn't a good substitute as it yields a different texture. Make sure to buy *sustainable* palm shortening.

Plantains Plantains are similar to bananas, but can't be swapped 1:1. Green plantains are starchier, and ripened yellow/black plantains are sweeter and used for baked goods. You can find plantains in many health food stores and Latin American grocery stores.

Sweet potatoes Sweet potatoes come in several varieties, and many are used in this cookbook. Each recipe notes the variety used as well as a substitute, if applicable.

Tapioca starch Tapioca starch is also derived from the yucca plant and is used in baked goods. Though it can often be swapped 1:1 with arrowroot starch in baked goods, I would not swap it in savory meals as it can produce a gummy texture.

Tigernut flour Tigernuts are not nuts, but tubers! Tigernut flour has a similar texture to almond flour, but is slightly starchier, which makes it great for baked goods. You can find tigernuts and tigernut flour online or in many health food stores.

GADGETS & COOKWARE GUIDE

Adding new recipes to your rotation can often mean adding new gadgets and cookware to your kitchen. Most cookware in this section is standard in most kitchens. However, you don't need to run out and buy every single item to be successful. Go at your pace and add new items slowly.

Baking sheet Also known as a cookie sheet, you'll want to have a few of these on hand so you can make multiple dishes at once. Stainless steel or ceramic are both great options.

Casserole dishes and a brownie pan Ceramic casserole dishes are a must for making classic recipes such as Sloppy Joe Casserole (page 110) and Tuna Zoodle Casserole (page 152). Having a 9 x 13-inch (23 x 33 cm) casserole dish on hand is best for large casseroles, but it's also a good idea to have smaller sizes if you wish to scale down any recipes. An 8 x 8-inch (20 x 20 cm) brownie pan can also be used for casseroles as well as crisps, dessert bars, and brownies.

Cheesecloth Cheesecloth is cost effective as it's reusable and is used in recipes such as Coconut Yogurt (page 37), and can be used to strain excess water from steamed vegetables.

Food processor A food processor is useful for shredding vegetables such as zucchini and sweet potatoes. If shredding is your goal rather than blending, I highly recommend using a food processor versus a blender as the two yield different results.

Glass storage containers When it comes to food storage, plastics are not a preferable choice as they can leech harmful chemicals into our food. Opt for glass for safer food storage.

Handheld milk frother This is the secret for making a perfect gelatin egg every time! You can find handheld milk frothers for $10 or less online.

High-speed blender A high-speed blender is helpful for making soups and sauces.

Immersion blender This tool is great for quickly blitzing soups or sauces.

Knives and other cooking utensils When it comes to cooking knives, you can do a lot with a good quality chef's knife. I also recommend a stainless steel spatula, soup ladle, large cooking spoon, whisk, serving spoon, and kitchen scissors.

Mandoline These are great for making chips! You can use a sharp knife if you don't have a mandoline, but these allow for a more consistently sliced end product. They're sold online and can often be found in the kitchen section of stores.

Meat thermometer A meat thermometer is essential to making sure your meat is perfectly cooked every time. Digital meat thermometers are inexpensive and readily available online and in many stores.

Mixing bowls I recommend having a few sizes of glass mixing bowls on hand.

Nut milk bag Nut milk bags are inexpensive and incredibly convenient to have around. You can buy these online and often at health food stores, or you can buy these online and often uses cheesecloth for many recipes that call for a nut milk bag.

Parchment paper (unbleached) Unbleached parchment is untreated and safer to cook with than bleached.

Pots and pans When it comes to cookware, I always recommend cast iron pans, as well as enamel-coated Dutch ovens whenever possible. They're easy to clean and are a safer option than nonstick. Stainless steel is another great option for cookware.

Slow cooker A slow cooker, or electric pressure cooker with a slow cooker function, is a great addition to your kitchen for making cooking less hands on.

Spiralizer These tools are perfect for making vegetable noodles. I highly recommend investing in a larger spiralizer with multiple blades.

Waffle maker There are myriad waffle makers on the market that would work for this cookbook. Every waffle maker is different, so there's a bit of a learning curve to making them perfect.

A FEW NOTES ON . . .

Oven cook time Cook times vary from oven to oven. If it's your first time making a recipe, keep an eye on it to ensure it doesn't burn, overcook, or undercook. I often set my timer for 5 to 8 minutes less than the suggested cook time to properly gauge cook time for my own oven.

Seasoning with salt Salt is different to every palate. It's best to add salt while cooking to build flavor, but if you need to add more or less salt than a recipe says, trust your palate and adjust accordingly.

Reheating food Several recipes in this book are labeled as meal-prep ready, which means they're great for storing and serving later. Reheating can often be done in a pan on the stovetop for about 2 minutes, under the broiler in the oven, or in a toaster oven. If you are away from a stove or oven, I recommend getting a desk slow cooker that only heats food, or a small portable oven, such as those made by Hot Logic. These are both available on Amazon and although they don't cook food, they do a wonderful job of reheating!

ICONS GUIDE

You'll spot the following icons throughout this book:

 Coconut free: Although coconut products are AIP compliant, coconut intolerance is common. This icon indicates coconut-free recipes.

 Meal-prep ready: This highlights recipes that are great for simple meal preparation. Make one of these meals on the weekend and store it in separate serving-size containers to enjoy throughout the week.

 One pan: This icon is for whole meals easily made in one pan or pot for easier cleanup!

 Under 45 minutes: These recipes can be made in less than 45 minutes—from start to finish.

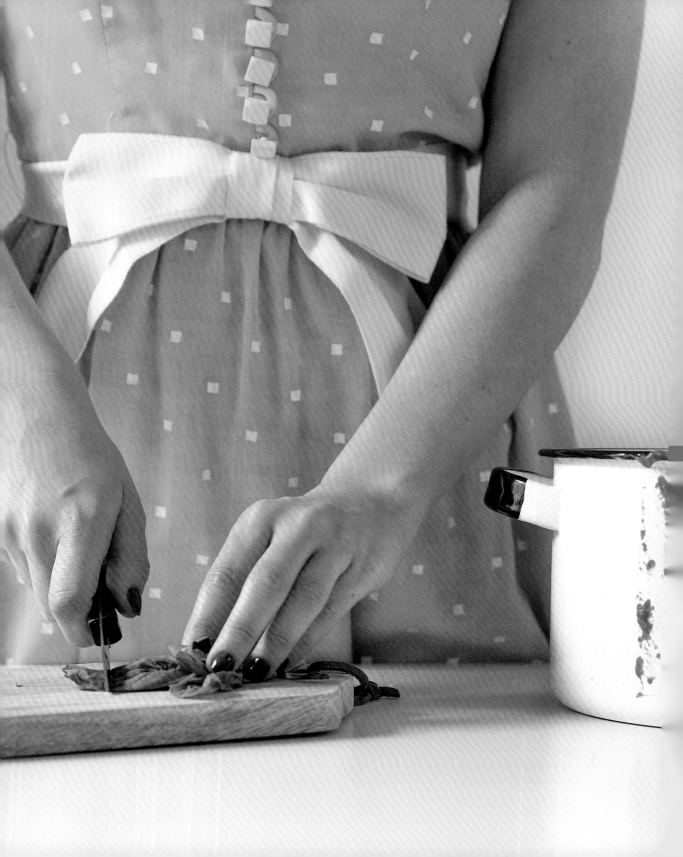

CHAPTER 2

AIP BASICS

When following the autoimmune protocol, it can be difficult to find compliant basics that are premade. Gone are the days of popping into the grocery store on the way home from work to grab a jar of pasta sauce and go on your way. Does that mean the days of enjoying pasta sauce, ketchup, and cheese are gone? Of course not! You can easily make these basics autoimmune protocol compliant and keep them on hand for when you need them.

BEEF BONE BROTH

Beef Bone Broth is full of gut-healing collagen and minerals such as calcium, magnesium, and more! It's rich, nourishing, and perfect for making stews and pot roasts.

STOVETOP   **PREP TIME** 20 min   **COOK TIME** 12 to 24 hours
SLOW COOKER   **PREP TIME** 20 min   **COOK TIME** 24 hours
YIELD Makes 6 to 8 servings

2 pounds (900 g) meaty
soup bones

2 pounds (900 g) mixed joint
bones (knuckle, neck, etc.)

2 celery stalks,
roughly chopped

2 carrots, roughly chopped

1 onion, peeled and quartered

2 tablespoons (8 g) chopped
fresh parsley

3 garlic cloves, chopped

3 bay leaves

½ teaspoon sea salt

1 tablespoon (15 ml) apple
cider vinegar

STOVETOP

1. Preheat the oven to 350°F (180°C, or gas mark 4) and line a baking sheet with parchment paper.

2. Place the bones on the prepared baking sheet and roast for 15 minutes. Using tongs, transfer the bones to a large stockpot and place the pot over low heat.

3. Add the remaining ingredients and enough water to cover everything. Cover the pot and bring the liquid to a very low simmer. Simmer for at least 12 hours or, ideally, 24 hours.

4. Strain the broth and let cool. Refrigerate in a glass container for three to four days or keep frozen for three to four months.

SLOW COOKER

1. Preheat the oven to 350°F (180°C, or gas mark 4). Line a baking sheet with parchment paper.

2. Place the bones on the prepared baking sheet and roast for 15 minutes. Using tongs, transfer the bones to a slow cooker. Place the remaining ingredients on top and add enough water to cover everything. Cover the slow cooker, set it to low, and cook for 24 hours.

3. Strain the broth and let cool. Refrigerate in a glass container for three to four days or keep frozen for three to four months.

CHICKEN BONE BROTH

Chicken Bone Broth is a more neutral-tasting broth than Beef Bone Broth (see previous page) and is great for sipping in a mug on its own or adding to chicken soups and sauces. Oh, and don't let the chicken feet scare you—they add tons of healing collagen that your gut will thank you for.

STOVETOP   **PREP TIME:** 20 minutes   **COOK TIME:** 12 to 24 hours
SLOW COOKER   **PREP TIME:** 20 minutes   **COOK TIME:** 24 hours

YIELD Makes 6 to 8 servings

1 chicken carcass, meat removed

4 to 6 chicken feet, washed and nails removed (see Notes)

2 celery stalks, roughly chopped

2 carrots, roughly chopped

1 onion, peeled and quartered

2 tablespoons (8 g) chopped fresh parsley

3 bay leaves

½ teaspoon sea salt

1 tablespoon (15 ml) apple cider vinegar

STOVETOP

1. In a large stockpot over low heat, combine all the ingredients and add enough water to cover everything. Cover the pot and bring the liquid to a very low simmer. Simmer for at least 8 hours or up to 24 hours.

2. Strain the broth and let cool. Refrigerate in a glass container for three to four days or keep frozen for three to four months.

SLOW COOKER

1. In a slow cooker, combine all the ingredients and add enough water to cover everything. Cover the slow cooker, set it to low, and cook for 24 hours.

2. Strain the broth and let cool. Refrigerate in a glass container for three to four days or keep frozen for three to four months.

NOTES

You can find chicken feet at the butcher's counter or farmer's markets. Wash them well and use a sharp, sturdy knife to remove the toenails!

GELATIN EGG

Egg-free baking doesn't have to be a chore. Gelatin eggs are my favorite egg substitute in baked goods, and they add a healing boost. Gelatin and collagen are both found in the bones and cartilage of animals; gelatin is simply the cooked version of collagen. Both have anti-inflammatory properties. Gelatin eggs are perfect for making gelatinous recipes such as Orange Turmeric Gummies (page 184) and others. Make the gelatin egg *immediately* before using—if left to sit it will not work in the recipe.

PREP TIME 5 minutes   **COOK TIME** 5 minutes   **YIELD** Makes 1 gelatin egg

¼ cup (60 ml) water

1 tablespoon (7 g)
grass-fed gelatin

1. Place the water in a small saucepan. Slowly pour in the gelatin. Using a fork, gently mix, breaking up any clumps. Let bloom for 2 to 3 minutes until the mixture hardens.

2. Place the pan over low heat. Cook for 60 to 90 seconds to slowly melt the gelatin. Immediately remove from the heat once the gelatin melts and the mixture returns to liquid form.

3. Vigorously whisk the liquid until frothy. A milk frother speeds up the process and yields a perfectly frothy mixture.

4. Use the gelatin egg *immediately* in baking recipes.

NOTES

Collagen *cannot* be substituted for gelatin as it will not gel.

GRANDMA'S KRAUT

Sauerkraut is a great way to add fermented foods to your diet to support your gut health. It's simple to make at home and can be eaten as a side dish or used as a condiment.

PREP TIME 20 minutes   **FERMENTING TIME** 3 days   **YIELD** Makes 3 to 4 cups

1 medium (about 2 pounds, or 900 g) green cabbage, outer leaves removed and thoroughly washed

1½ teaspoons sea salt

1. Prepare a clean workstation and thoroughly clean a 1- to 2-quart (946 ml to 1.9 L) lidded glass jar.

2. Using a sharp knife, slice the cabbage into thin, even slices and remove the tough inner core. Transfer to a large, clean bowl and add the salt. Using your clean hands, squeeze the cabbage and work in the salt, like you're kneading dough. Continue for 5 to 10 minutes or until the cabbage releases liquid.

3. Place the cabbage in the clean glass jar and pack it down tightly. You want about 2 inches (5 cm) of space between the cabbage and the top of the jar.

4. Place a clean weight (such as a glass fermentation weight) into either a smaller jar or plastic bag and place it into the jar to weigh down the cabbage. Cover the jar with a clean cloth and set in a cool, dry place away from sunlight to ferment.

5. Watch the jar over the next four days to ensure the cabbage remains submerged in the brine. Push down the weight, if necessary.

6. After three or four days, use a clean wooden spoon to remove some of the cabbage for tasting. If you want to ferment it longer, return the weight to the jar and re-cover it with the cloth. Test daily until it reaches your desired flavor. Remove the weight, add the lid, and keep refrigerated for up to six months.

NOTES

Keep your work station as clean as possible to avoid unfriendly bacteria. You can also use other cabbage varieties, such as red cabbage.

BASIC CAULIFLOWER RICE

Cauliflower rice is easy to make and is the perfect substitute for rice! I use it in a variety of recipes in this book, or you can just serve it as a simple side dish for a protein.

PREP TIME 15 minutes   **COOK TIME** 10 minutes   **YIELD** Makes 2 servings

1 large head cauliflower, washed well and cut into florets

2 tablespoons (28 ml) avocado oil

½ teaspoon sea salt

1. In a food processor, process the cauliflower until it has a rice-like texture.

2. In a sauté pan over medium heat, heat the avocado oil.

3. Add the cauliflower rice and salt to the pan. Sauté for 5 to 8 minutes, stirring occasionally, or until the cauliflower rice is softened and cooked.

NOTES

For recipes that call for uncooked riced cauliflower, such as Shrimp & Grits with Spinach (page 148) or and Margherita Pizza (page 156), use the riced cauliflower as is after step 1.

CAULIFLOWER "CHEESE"

Cheese is one of those beloved foods that can keep us from fully committing to a dairy-free lifestyle! Although nut milk cheese is growing in popularity, it doesn't leave much room for those who are both dairy and nut free. This cauliflower "cheese" saves the day!

PREP TIME 20 minutes   **CHILLING TIME** 10 minutes   **YIELD** Makes 5 to 6 servings

2 cups (200 g) cauliflower, steamed

¼ cup (30 g) tapioca starch

3 tablespoons (45 ml) avocado oil

3 tablespoons (11.5 g) nutritional yeast

3 tablespoons (21 g) gelatin

1 teaspoon apple cider vinegar

½ teaspoon sea salt

1. Neatly line a small glass storage container or small loaf pan with parchment paper. (I use a round, 2-cup, or 475 ml, container to make a cheese wheel.) Alternately, use a silicone mold of your desired shape. Set aside.

2. In a food processor, combine the hot cauliflower with the remaining ingredients and blend until smooth and fully incorporated. Pour the cheese mixture into the prepared vessel and smooth the top with a rubber spatula or the back of a spoon. Refrigerate for at least 3 hours to chill and harden.

3. Remove from the mold. If there are any dents in the cheese, use your clean fingers to smooth them out. Slice to serve with recipes such as the Charcuterie Board with Crackers and Artichoke Hummus (page 48).

NIGHTSHADE-FREE KETCHUP

I am a *huge* ketchup enthusiast. I put ketchup on everything when I was a kid and missed it dearly when I first went nightshade free. This nightshade-free ketchup tastes just like the real deal without any tomato or corn syrup.

PREP TIME 10 minutes   **COOK TIME** 40 minutes   **YIELD** Makes 1½ cups (500 g)

2 cups (260 g) chopped carrot

⅓ cup (75 g) chopped beet

1 tablespoon (15 ml) avocado oil

1 medium onion, chopped

⅓ cup (81 g) sliced no-sugar-added canned pear

2 tablespoons (28 ml) fresh lemon juice

1 tablespoon (20 g) maple syrup

1 teaspoon apple cider vinegar

2 teaspoons garlic powder

½ teaspoon sea salt, plus more as needed

1. In a medium saucepan, combine the carrot, beet, and enough water to cover. Place the pan over medium heat and bring to a low simmer. Cook for 25 to 30 minutes or until the vegetables are fork-tender. Strain the water and set the carrot and beet aside to cool.

2. In a skillet over medium heat, heat the avocado oil.

3. Add the onion and sauté for 3 to 4 minutes until translucent. Transfer to a high-speed blender.

4. Add the cooked carrot and beet mixture and the remaining ingredients. Blend until completely smooth. Transfer to an airtight container and refrigerate until chilled.

5. Taste and season with more salt, if desired. Refrigerate in a glass container for three to four days or keep frozen for three to four months.

NOTES

Freeze the ketchup in small batches to have on hand for recipes, as needed.

NIGHTSHADE-FREE "TOMATO" SAUCE

Growing up in an Italian-American family, my dad used to say spaghetti sauce ran through his veins! Ditto. However, when I finally realized how inflammatory nightshades where for me, I didn't know what to do. This nightshade-free "tomato" sauce has all the flavor we grew up loving in a classic marinara, but without the tomato!

PREP TIME 15 minutes   **COOK TIME** 40 minutes   **YIELD** Makes 6 cups (1.5 L)

2 tablespoons (28 ml) olive oil

2 garlic cloves, minced

1 white onion, diced

2½ cups (325 g) chopped carrot

1¼ cups (125 g) chopped celery

1¼ cups (281 g) chopped beet

1⅓ cups (315 ml) water

1 tablespoon (3 g) fresh basil leaves (optional)

2 teaspoons chopped fresh parsley

1 teaspoon dried oregano

½ teaspoon sea salt

2 tablespoons (28 ml) fresh lemon juice

1. In a large deep saucepan over low heat, heat the olive oil.

2. Add the garlic and onion and sauté for 3 to 4 minutes until the onion is translucent.

3. Add the carrot, celery, and beet and sauté for 18 to 20 minutes or until tender.

4. Add the water, basil (if using), parsley, oregano, and salt to the pan and bring to a low simmer. Cover the pan and simmer for 10 minutes. Remove from the heat, keeping the pot covered, and let cool slightly.

5. Carefully spoon the vegetables and cooking liquid into a blender. Add the lemon juice. Blend for 20 to 30 seconds or until smooth.

NOTES

This sauce is used in several recipes in this book. For a more neutral tasting sauce, omit the basil. I recommend freezing this sauce in small batches of 1 to 2 cups (250 to 500 g) to have on hand whenever you need it.

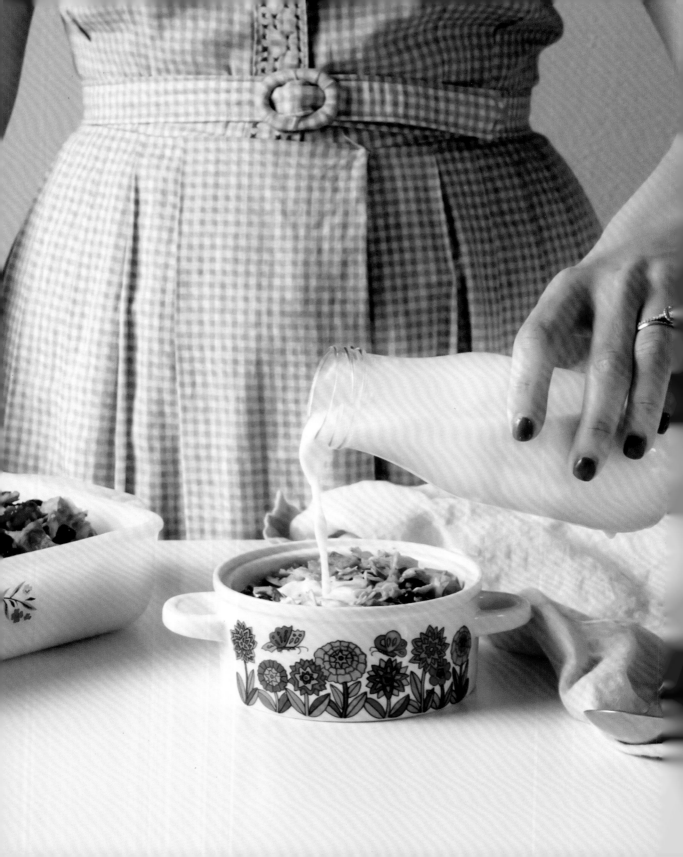

CHAPTER 3

BREAKFAST IN BED

How in the world do you enjoy breakfast without eggs and grains? That's a question I asked myself years ago and one people often ask me when they learn the AIP doesn't include either of these foods. We're conditioned to believe breakfast is an incredibly narrow meal with only a few options allowed. There is so much more to breakfast than *just* eggs and oatmeal.

These recipes allow you to get creative while still paying homage to comfort-food classics such as bagels and lox and French toast. Remember to keep an open mind—what you wind up trying and liking may surprise you!

← Apple Cinnamon Granola with Coconut Milk, page 38

BLUEBERRY WAFFLES

There's nothing quite like waffles on the weekend, right? You don't need to buy a box of frozen waffles or go to a diner. All you need is a waffle maker and the following ingredients to make this classic, comforting, AIP-compliant breakfast.

PREP TIME 10 minutes   **COOK TIME** 25 minutes   **YIELD** Makes 3 to 4 waffles

1 cup (140 g) cassava flour

¼ cup (36 g) arrowroot starch

3 tablespoons (21 g) tigernut flour

2 tablespoons (10 g) collagen powder

1 teaspoon ground cinnamon

¾ teaspoon baking soda

¼ teaspoon sea salt

¼ cup (56 g) coconut oil, melted, plus more for the waffle maker

¼ cup (80 g) maple syrup, plus more for topping (optional)

2 cups (475 ml) coconut milk

1 teaspoon apple cider vinegar

Fresh blueberries, for topping

1. In a large bowl, stir together the cassava flour, arrowroot starch, tigernut flour, collagen powder, cinnamon, baking soda, and salt.

2. Add the coconut oil and maple syrup and stir to combine.

3. Stir in the coconut milk and vinegar, stirring until fully combined.

4. Coat the waffle iron with the coconut oil and preheat it according to the manufacturer's instructions.

5. Pour one-fourth to one-third of the batter into the waffle iron. Close and cook per the manufacturer's instruction until the waffle is golden brown. Using tongs or a fork, carefully remove the waffle. Repeat with the remaining batter. Serve the waffles topped with fresh blueberries and maple syrup, if desired.

Also pictured, Apple Chicken Sausage, page 39 →

NOTES

Waffle iron cook times vary. Keep an eye on your waffles to ensure they don't over- or undercook.

For crispier waffles, don't stack the cooked waffles on top of each another or the heat and moisture will soften them. Make sure they're not touching or keep them on separate plates.

If you freeze the waffles, defrost them overnight in the refrigerator and re-crisp them in a skillet.

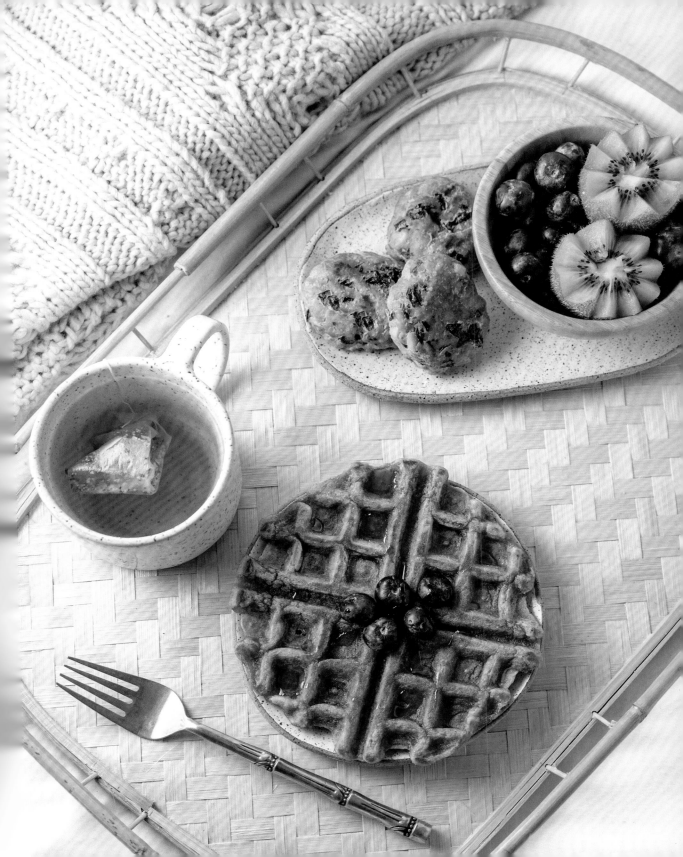

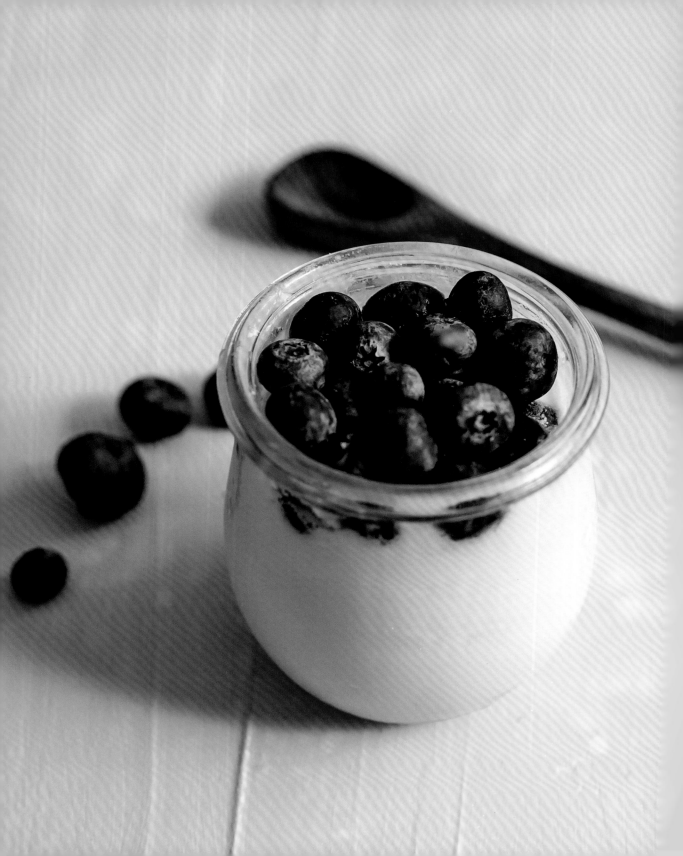

COCONUT YOGURT

Yogurt is a delicious breakfast option when paired with something like Apple Chicken Sausage (page 39), or used in a variety of other ways. It's easy to make your own coconut yogurt at home, and it is a great way to add more beneficial bacteria to your diet! If you'd like more than one serving, simply double the recipe.

PREP TIME 10 minutes   **FERMENTING TIME** 26 hours   **YIELD** Makes 1 serving

1½ cup (360 g) coconut cream

2 teaspoons tapioca starch

2 probiotic capsules

1 to 2 teaspoons honey (optional)

3 tablespoons (weight varies) fresh berries, plus more for

topping (optional)

1. Place the coconut cream in a clean glass jar or bowl and stir until it's no longer solid, but creamy.

2. Stir in the tapioca starch and mix well to break up any clumps.

3. Break open the probiotic capsules and use a small wooden spoon to gently stir the contents into the yogurt.

4. Place a piece of cheesecloth over the yogurt mixture and let sit on the counter, out of the sun and away from extreme heat or cold, for 24 hours.

5. Remove the cheesecloth and refrigerate the yogurt for 1 to 2 hours to chill.

6. Stir in the honey (if using) and serve topped with the berries (if using).

NOTES

For the probiotic capsules, use a high-quality probiotic that is not soil based and does not contain prebiotics, dairy, or other fillers.

Depending on the kind of coconut cream you use, this yogurt may solidify in the refrigerator. Place it on the counter for 30 minutes before serving or add it to a blender with 1 to 2 tablespoons (15 to 28 ml) of coconut milk and blend to make it creamy again.

APPLE CINNAMON GRANOLA WITH COCONUT MILK

Cereal and milk are a classic! This is a great breakfast for special occasions when paired with a protein such as Apple Chicken Sausage (opposite page), or enjoy it as a simple after-school or—after-work snack.

PREP TIME 10 minutes   **COOK TIME** 15 minutes   **YIELD** Makes 4 servings

FOR THE COCONUT MILK

4 cups (966 ml) water

2 cups (160 g) shredded unsweetened coconut

2 teaspoons maple syrup (optional)

FOR THE APPLE CINNAMON GRANOLA

1½ cups (90 g) coconut chips

½ cup (30 g) baked apple chips

½ cup (45 g) sliced tigernuts

¼ cup (40 g) sugar- and oil-free dried cranberries

3 tablespoons (42 g) coconut oil, melted

2 tablespoons (40 g) maple syrup

½ teaspoon ground cinnamon

1. To make the coconut milk: In a medium saucepan over medium heat, heat the water until very hot, but not boiling. Carefully transfer to a high-speed blender and add the coconut. Blend for 2 minutes on medium speed.

2. Using cheesecloth or a nut milk bag, strain the coconut milk into a bowl. Stir in the maple syrup (if using). Let the milk cool before transferring to an airtight container and refrigerating for two to three days. If the coconut milk separates, use a blender to reincorporate the cream and water.

3. To make the apple cinnamon granola: Preheat the oven to 350°F (180°C, or gas mark 4) and line a large baking sheet with parchment paper. Set aside.

4. In a large bowl, combine the coconut chips and apple chips. Using a large spoon, lightly crush them into smaller pieces.

5. Add the remaining ingredients and mix well. Pour the granola mixture onto the prepared baking sheet and bake for 8 to 10 minutes.

6. Let cool before serving with coconut milk or eating as a snack by itself. Keep leftovers refrigerated in a glass container for three to four days.

NOTES

Keep the coconut milk and cream on hand to make recipes such as Ranch Dip (page 139) or Coconut Yogurt (page 37).

APPLE CHICKEN SAUSAGE

Store-bought sausages are typically made with fillers, artificial sugars, and nightshade spices that aren't AIP compliant. Happily, they're quite simple to make at home. These sausage patties are the perfect filling breakfast to add to your rotation.

PREP TIME 10 minutes   **COOK TIME** 30 minutes   **YIELD** Makes 10 to 12 sausages

1 pound (455 g) ground chicken or turkey

1 cup (30 g) spinach, chopped

½ cup (75 g) finely diced peeled apple

2 tablespoons (28 g) coconut oil

2 teaspoons dried sage

1 teaspoon dried thyme

¾ teaspoon sea salt

1. Preheat the oven to 375°F (190°C, or gas mark 5) and line a baking sheet with parchment paper. Set aside.

2. In a large bowl, combine all the ingredients and stir to mix thoroughly. Roll the mixture into 10 to 12 small, flattened sausage patties about 2 inches (5 cm) in diameter. Place the patties on the prepared baking sheet. Bake for 25 to 30 minutes, flipping the sausages halfway through the baking time, or until the internal temperature reaches 165°F (74°C) on a meat thermometer. Remove from the oven and serve warm.

NOTES

To enjoy throughout the week, refrigerate in a covered glass container for up to three days.

BANANA BREAD FRENCH TOAST

French toast isn't exactly the most nutrient-dense breakfast in the world. In reality, it's much more of a treat or dessert. However, sometimes it's just what we're craving or perfect for special occasions. This French toast is made from homemade banana bread and an egg-free French toast batter. Top it all off with maple syrup and banana slices, and you've got one decadent AIP-friendly French toast!

PREP TIME 20 minutes, plus overnight chilling   **COOK TIME** 1 hour   **YIELD** Makes 8 to 9 servings

FOR THE BANANA BREAD

3 tablespoons (42 g) coconut oil, plus more for preparing the loaf pan

½ cup (56 g) coconut flour

¼ cup (35 g) cassava flour

¼ cup (30 g) tapioca starch

2 tablespoons (18 g) coconut sugar

1 teaspoon ground cinnamon

¾ teaspoon baking soda

2 yellow plantains with black spots, peeled

2 very ripe bananas, peeled

FOR THE FRENCH TOAST BATTER

½ cup (120 ml) coconut milk

1 tablespoon (7 g) coconut flour

½ teaspoon ground cinnamon

2 to 4 tablespoons (28 to 56 g) coconut oil, plus more as needed

FOR SERVING

1 banana, sliced

2 to 3 tablespoons (40 to 60 g) maple syrup

1. To make the banana bread: Preheat the oven to 375°F (190°C, or gas mark 5). Line a 9 x 5-inch (23 x 13 cm) loaf pan with parchment paper and lightly coat it with coconut oil.

2. In a large bowl, stir together the coconut and cassava flours, the tapioca starch, coconut sugar, cinnamon, and baking soda. Set aside.

3. In a food processor, combine the plantains and bananas. Thoroughly process until completely mashed. Scoop out the plantain mixture and transfer to a medium bowl. Add the coconut oil and mix well. Add the wet ingredients to the dry ingredients and mix until combined. Pour the batter into the prepared loaf pan and smooth the top with a rubber spatula or the back of a spoon. Bake for 40 to 45 minutes.

4. Remove and let cool completely. Cover and refrigerate overnight before making the French toast. Cut into eight or nine slices when cooled.

5. To make the French toast: In a small bowl, whisk the coconut milk, coconut flour, and cinnamon. Set aside.

6. In a medium skillet over medium-low heat, melt the coconut oil.

7. Working with one to three slices of banana bread at a time, dip them into the French toast batter, evenly coating both sides. Place the slices into the skillet and cook for about 2 minutes per side or until slightly crispy. Transfer to a plate and repeat the process, adding more coconut oil, if needed. If the skillet gets dirty between batches, wipe it out and add fresh coconut oil.

8. To serve: Top the French toast with banana slices and maple syrup.

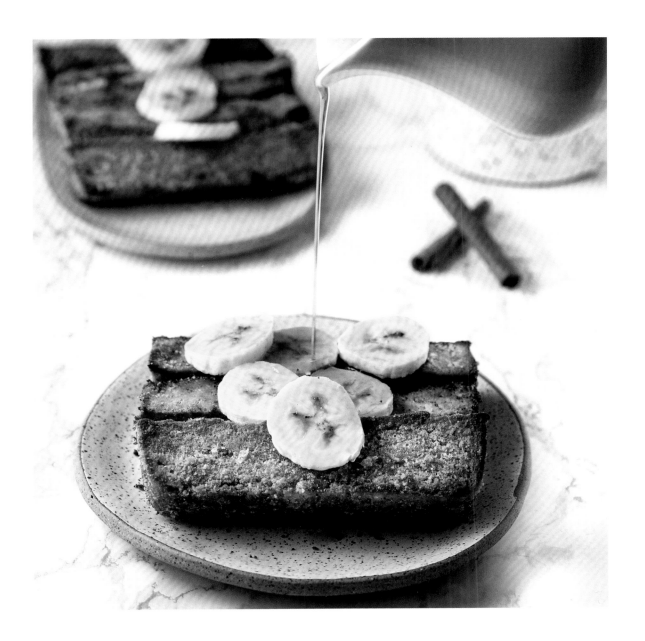

NOTES

This French toast is better when the banana bread has more time to sit, so make it the day before and refrigerate overnight before making the French toast.

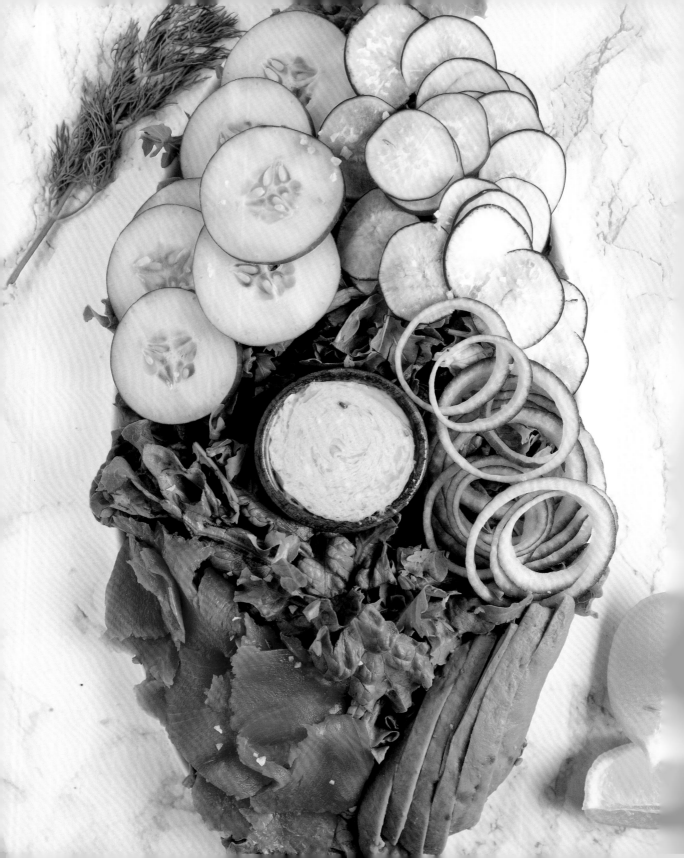

HOLD-THE-BAGEL LOX BREAKFAST SALAD WITH CREAM "CHEESE" DRESSING

Are you craving bagels for breakfast? You can have your bagel without actually *eating* the bagel with this breakfast salad! With all the yummy everything bagel toppings and a cream "cheese" dressing, you won't even miss the bagel. This breakfast salad is perfect for brunch where everyone can help themselves!

PREP TIME 25 minutes   **YIELD** Makes 2 to 3 servings

FOR THE SALAD

4 to 5 cups (144 to 180 g) green leaf lettuce, chopped

8 to 12 ounces (225 to 340 g) smoked salmon

1 cucumber, thinly sliced

2 or 3 radishes, thinly sliced

½ red onion, thinly sliced

½ avocado, pitted, peeled, and sliced

1 tablespoon (4 g) chopped fresh dill

1 teaspoon toasted onion flakes

FOR THE CREAM "CHEESE" DRESSING

¼ cup (60 g) coconut cream

1 tablespoon (15 ml) avocado oil

1 teaspoon apple cider vinegar

1 teaspoon nutritional yeast

2 teaspoons chopped fresh chives

½ teaspoon toasted onion flakes

¼ teaspoon sea salt

1. To make the salad: Assemble the salad on a large serving platter by starting with the lettuce and then layering the rest of the ingredients on top. Either separate the ingredients so they look visually pleasing or toss them together, as you prefer.

2. To make the dressing: In a small bowl, combine all the ingredients. Whisk until creamy. Serve the dressing on the side or drizzled over the salad.

TURKEY AND CARROT BREAKFAST HASH

Shredded carrots make an excellent substitute for the traditional potato in hash browns! This breakfast hash is filling, nutrient dense, and simple to make.

PREP TIME 10 minutes   **COOK TIME** 25 minutes   **YIELD** Makes 4 servings

3 bacon slices, chopped

1 pound (455 g) ground turkey

½ teaspoon sea salt, divided

3 cups (330 g) shredded carrot

1 leek, cleaned well, white part cut into half-moons

1 cup (67 g) chopped stemmed kale

2 teaspoons fresh rosemary leaves, chopped

1 teaspoon dried sage

1. In a large deep skillet over medium heat, cook the bacon for 6 to 8 minutes or until crispy. Remove the bacon from the pan and set aside, leaving about 1 tablespoon (15 ml) of bacon fat in the skillet to cook the ground turkey. Return the skillet to the heat.

2. Season the ground turkey with ¼ teaspoon of salt and place it in the skillet. Brown the turkey for 5 minutes, breaking it up with the back of a spoon, or until fully cooked. Remove and set aside, leaving about 2 tablespoons (28 ml) of fat in the skillet. Return the skillet to the heat.

3. Add the shredded carrot and cook for 5 to 6 minutes or until softened and lightly browned.

4. Stir in the leek, kale, rosemary, sage, and the remaining ¼ teaspoon of salt. Cook for 3 to 4 minutes to soften the leeks and kale.

5. Reincorporate the turkey and bacon and sauté for another minute to reheat. Serve warm.

NOTES

Save time by using a bag of already shredded carrots. Portion the hash into individual glass containers to enjoy for breakfasts throughout the week.

BREAKFAST TACO BOWLS

Are you craving something hearty for breakfast? These breakfast taco bowls are just the thing! They're made without eggs, nightshades, beans, or a taco shell, but have all the flavors of a taco.

PREP TIME 5 minutes   **COOK TIME** 20 minutes   **YIELD** Makes 4 servings

1 pound (455 g) ground beef

1 teaspoon sea salt, divided

2 teaspoons garlic powder, divided

2 tablespoons (2 g) cilantro, chopped and divided

2 tablespoons (15 ml) avocado oil

3 to 4 cups (141 to 188 g) torn romaine lettuce leaves

1 yellow plantain, peeled and diced, or sweet potato

3 or 4 radishes, thinly sliced

½ red onion, sliced

Guacamole (page 59), or 1 or 2 avocados, pitted, peeled, and sliced

Lime wedges, for serving

1. In a large skillet over medium heat, brown the ground beef. While browning, stir in ½ teaspoon of salt, 1 teaspoon of garlic powder, and 1 tablespoon (1 g) of cilantro. Once browned, remove the mixture from the pan and set aside, discarding the fat.

2. Return the skillet to medium heat and add the avocado oil and plantain. Season with the remaining ½ teaspoon of salt and 1 teaspoon of garlic powder. Cook for 6 to 8 minutes or until softened.

3. Assemble the bowls by starting with the romaine lettuce. Add a layer of beef, plantain, radish, and red onion. Top with guacamole or avocado slices and sprinkle with the remaining 1 tablespoon (1 g) of cilantro. Serve with the lime wedges for squeezing.

NOTES

To make this meal-prep ready, portion the breakfast taco bowls into separate glass storage containers, separating the romaine lettuce to keep it crisp. Omit the guacamole and instead serve with fresh avocado.

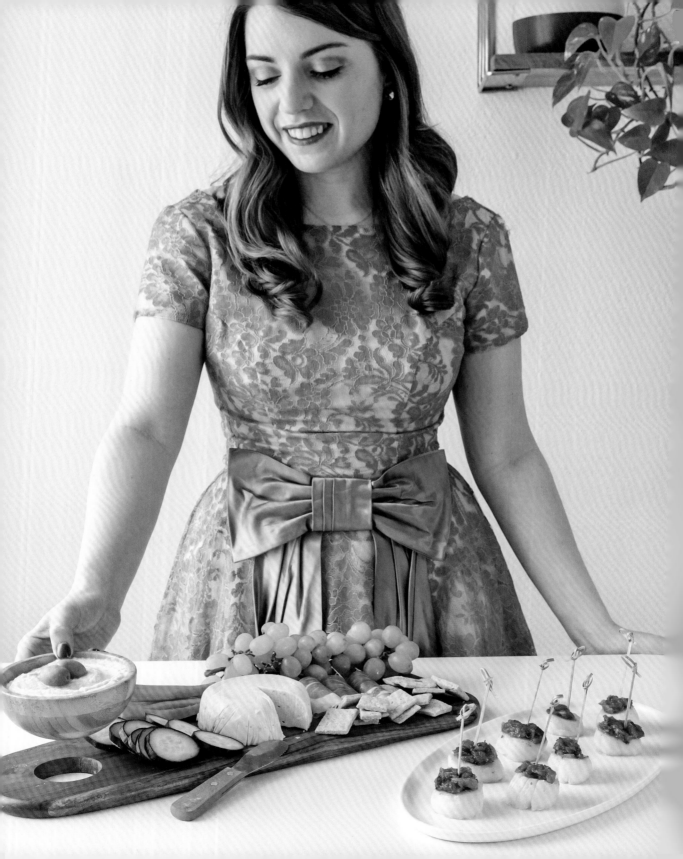

CHAPTER 4

APPETIZERS, DIPS & SNACKS

Snacks, dips, and appetizers don't have to come from a bag or container and be super-processed to be delicious. Not even close! Snacks made at home can be far more flavorful.

These recipes are perfect for pleasing a party crowd, keeping to yourself on movie night, or taking to work.

← Charcuterie Board with Crackers and Artichoke Hummus, page 48 and Scallops with Bacon Jam, page 54

CHARCUTERIE BOARD WITH CRACKERS AND ARTICHOKE HUMMUS

Charcuterie boards are an easy way to please and impress party guests! Now, you'll also mystify guests when serving this charcuterie board that's free of dairy, legumes, and grains but *still* includes "cheese," crackers, and hummus. One look and guests will be asking how in the world you did it!

PREP TIME 30 minutes   **COOK TIME** 12 minutes   **YIELD** Makes 5 to 6 servings

FOR THE CRACKERS

¼ cup (56 g) coconut oil, plus more for preparing the baking sheet

1 cup (112 g) tigernut flour

¼ cup (36 g) arrowroot starch

1 teaspoon dried thyme

1 teaspoon dried rosemary

½ teaspoon sea salt

1 Gelatin Egg (page 26)

FOR THE ARTICHOKE HUMMUS

2 cups (600 g) artichoke hearts

3 tablespoons plus 1 teaspoon (50 ml) olive oil

Juice of 1 lemon

1 garlic clove

1 tablespoon (4 g) chopped fresh parsley

½ teaspoon sea salt

2 or 3 green olives

FOR THE BOARD

Cauliflower "Cheese" (page 29)

3 or 4 carrots, sliced

1 cucumber, sliced

5 or 6 radishes

3 or 4 slices prosciutto

Green or red grapes

1 apple, sliced

1. To make the crackers: Preheat the oven to 350°F (180°C, or gas mark 4) and line a baking sheet with parchment paper. Lightly coat it with 1 teaspoon of coconut oil.

2. In a large bowl, stir together the dry ingredients.

3. Add the coconut oil and stir to mix.

4. Prepare the Gelatin Egg and add it to the dough. Mix until fully incorporated. Transfer the dough to the prepared baking sheet and flatten it with your hands or place another piece of parchment on top and flatten it with a rolling pin until cracker thin. Slice with a pizza cutter or sharp knife into desired sizes. Bake for 10 to 12 minutes.

5. To make the artichoke hummus: In a food processor, combine the artichokes, 3 tablespoons (45 ml) of olive oil, the lemon juice, garlic, parsley, and salt. Process until smooth. Spoon the hummus into a small serving bowl and top with the olives and remaining 1 teaspoon of olive oil.

6. To assemble the board: Arrange all the ingredients on a large cutting board or serving platter. Serve fresh as an appetizer or party snack.

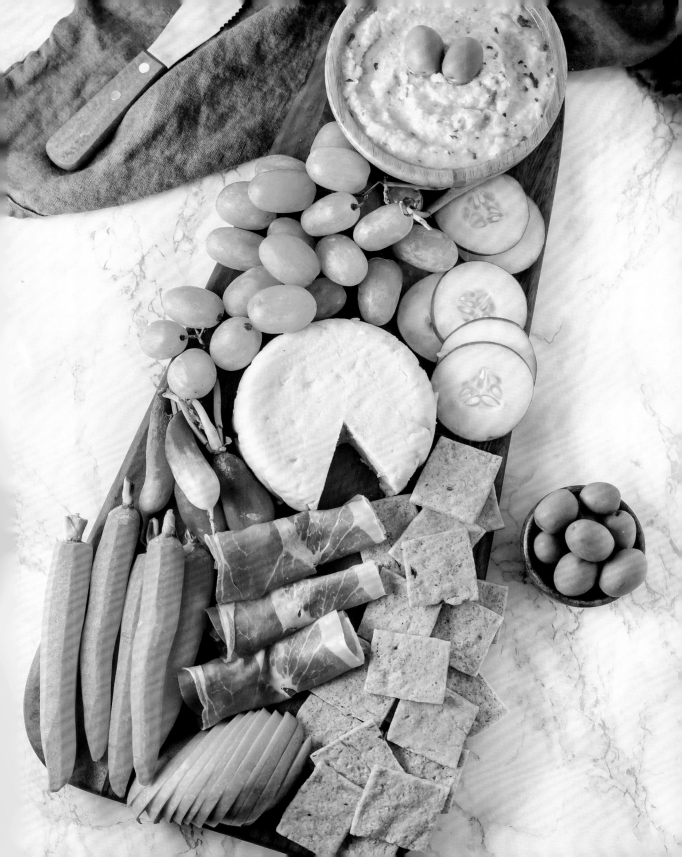

MINI-MEDITERRANEAN CHICKEN SKEWERS

I brought these chicken skewers to a baby shower and everyone loved them! They're the perfect filling finger food to serve when you want to satisfy your guests, but not cook an entire meal.

PREP TIME 45 minutes **COOK TIME** 20 minutes **YIELD** Makes 4 servings

1 pound (455 g) boneless chicken breast, cut into bite-size cubes

2 tablespoons (28 ml) avocado oil

Juice of ½ lemon

2 garlic cloves, minced

½ teaspoon sea salt

2 teaspoons chopped fresh parsley

1 teaspoon dried oregano

1 teaspoon dried basil

1 teaspoon onion powder

1. Soak several small bamboo skewers in water until ready to use.

2. In a medium bowl, combine the chicken, avocado oil, lemon juice, garlic, and seasonings. Gently stir to coat the chicken. Cover and refrigerate for 30 minutes to marinate.

3. Meanwhile, preheat the oven to 375°F (190°C, or gas mark 5) and line a baking sheet with parchment paper.

4. Remove the chicken mixture from the refrigerator and thread two to three pieces of chicken onto each bamboo skewer until all the pieces are used. Place the skewers on the prepared baking sheet. Bake for 15 to 20 minutes or until the chicken is cooked and the internal temperature reaches 165°F (74°C) on a meat thermometer. Serve and enjoy.

CHICKEN LIVER PÂTÉ

Chicken liver is much milder than beef liver and bursting with healing nutrients! Pâté is an easy way to get more liver into your diet, and it makes a great filling dip or snack along with sliced apples and carrots and even Plantain Chips (page 59). Be sure to use liver from pasture-raised chickens for the most nutrients!

PREP TIME 15 minutes   **COOK TIME** 15 minutes   **YIELD** Makes 4 servings

¼ cup (56 g) coconut oil, divided, plus more as needed

1 medium onion, diced

2 garlic cloves, minced

1 pound (455 g) chicken livers

½ teaspoon sea salt, plus more as needed

2 tablespoons (8 g) chopped fresh parsley, plus more as needed

2 teaspoons fresh rosemary leaves, chopped, chopped

1 teaspoon apple cider vinegar

FOR SERVING (OPTIONAL)

Apple slices

Carrot slices, for serving (optional)

Celery sticks, for serving (optional)

Plantain Chips (page 59), for serving (optional)

1. In a large sauté pan or skillet over medium heat, melt 2 tablespoons (28 g) of coconut oil.

2. Add the onion and garlic and sauté for 3 to 4 minutes until the onion is translucent.

3. Pat the chicken livers dry and season both sides with salt. Add them to the pan and sauté for 6 to 8 minutes or until browned on all sides. Add the parsley and rosemary to the pan and cook for 1 minute more. Transfer the mixture to a food processor.

4. Add the remaining 2 tablespoons (28 g) of coconut oil and the vinegar. Process until combined and creamy. Add more coconut oil, if needed, to get a texture you like.

5. Taste, adjust the seasoning, and serve with apple slices, carrot slices, celery sticks, or Plantain Chips (if using).

NOTES

To make this meal-prep ready, refrigerate it in individual glass containers for up to four days.

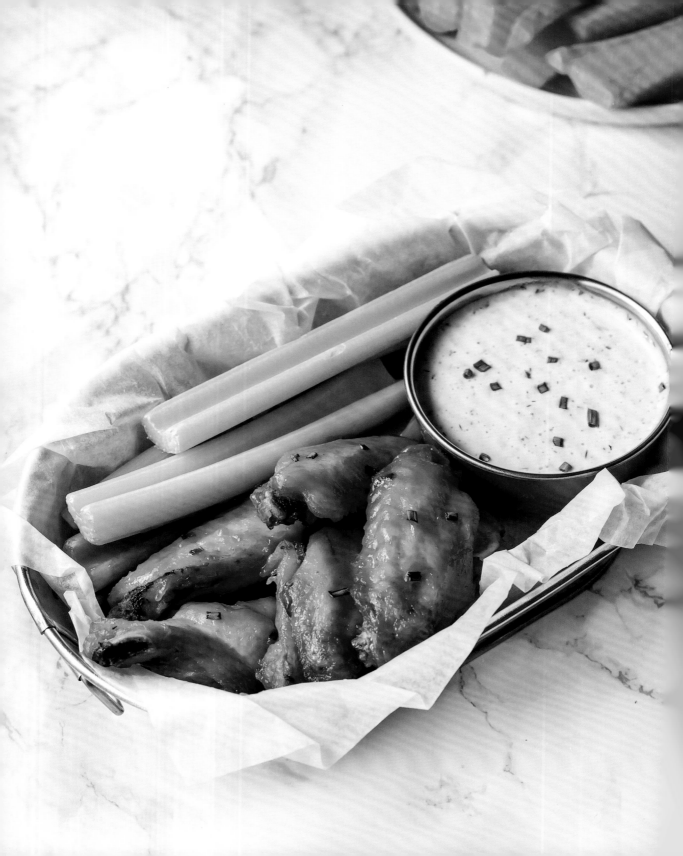

DAD'S FAVORITE BUFFALO CHICKEN WINGS

How in the world do you make buffalo wings AIP friendly? With a lot of determination and just a little magic in the kitchen! I shared this recipe with my parents, and my dad could not stop talking about it! This buffalo sauce is less spicy than one loaded with nightshade chile peppers, but it still satisfies the craving.

PREP TIME 15 minutes **COOK TIME** 1 hour **YIELD** Makes 2 to 3 servings

FOR THE BUFFALO SAUCE

3 tablespoons (45 g) coconut cream, softened

2 tablespoons (28 ml) coconut milk

2 tablespoons (31.5 g) Nightshade-Free "Tomato" Sauce (page 31; optional, see Notes)

2 tablespoons (28 ml) coconut aminos

1 tablespoon (20 g) honey

1 teaspoon onion powder

1 teaspoon garlic powder

1 teaspoon ground ginger

½ teaspoon ground turmeric

½ teaspoon smoked salt

1 to 3 teaspoons (2 to 7 g) horseradish powder

½ teaspoon arrowroot starch

FOR THE CHICKEN WINGS

1 pound (455 g) chicken wings

2 tablespoons (28 ml) avocado oil, or (28 g) coconut oil

½ teaspoon sea salt

2 teaspoons chopped fresh chives, plus more for garnishing

FOR SERVING

Ranch Dip (page 139)

Carrot sticks

Celery sticks

1. To make the buffalo sauce: In a small saucepan over low heat, combine the coconut cream, coconut milk, Nightshade-free "Tomato" Sauce, coconut aminos, honey, onion powder, garlic power, ginger, turmeric, and salt. Cook for 8 to 10 minutes, stirring occasionally.

2. One teaspoon at a time, stir in the horseradish powder and adjust to taste.

3. Whisk in the arrowroot starch. Cook for 1 to 2 minutes, stirring for to thicken the sauce. Set aside.

4. To make the chicken wings: Preheat the oven to 400°F (200°C, or gas mark 6) and line a baking sheet with parchment paper.

5. Place the chicken wings on the prepared baking sheet and drizzle with the avocado oil and salt. Bake for 30 minutes.

6. Let cool slightly before coating the wings with the buffalo sauce. Return to the oven and bake for 15 to 20 minutes more, or until the wings are cooked through.

7. Sprinkle with chives and serve with the ranch dip and carrot and celery sticks.

NOTES

Although optional, the "tomato" sauce adds extra flavor and color. If you prefer, use 1 tablespoon (15 ml) more coconut milk instead. For spicier wings, add more horseradish powder.

SCALLOPS WITH BACON JAM

Bacon-wrapped scallops are typical party fare but can get a little boring after a while. These bacon jam–topped scallops are a creative twist on a classic combination and every bit as delicious.

PREP TIME 10 minutes   **COOK TIME** 40 minutes   **YIELD** Makes 4 servings

FOR THE BACON JAM

3 bacon slices, chopped

1 medium yellow onion, diced

1 cup (178 g) dried dates, chopped

¾ cup (175 ml) water

¼ cup (60 ml) apple cider vinegar

2 tablespoons (40 g) maple syrup

Sea salt

FOR THE SCALLOPS

1 pound (455 g) sea scallops

¼ teaspoon sea salt

2 tablespoons (28 ml) avocado oil

1. To make the bacon jam: In a medium pot over medium heat, cook the bacon for 5 to 7 minutes or until lightly crispy. Using a slotted spoon, remove the bacon and set aside, leaving the fat in the pot. Return the pot to the heat.

2. Add the onion to the bacon fat and sauté for 5 to 6 minutes or until translucent.

3. Stir in the dates and use a fork to mash them into the onion. Sauté for about 3 minutes to soften.

4. Stir in the water, vinegar, maple syrup, and bacon. Bring to a low simmer and cook for 10 to 15 minutes, stirring often, until the bacon jam thickens. Taste and season with salt. Remove from the heat.

5. To make the scallops: Pat the scallops dry and lightly season both sides with salt.

6. In a medium sauté pan or skillet over medium-high heat, heat the avocado oil.

7. Add about half the scallops to the pan and sauté for 2 minutes on each side. Transfer to a serving plate. Repeat until all the scallops are seared.

8. Top each scallop with 1 to 2 tablespoons (15 to 30 g) of Bacon Jam. (The amount will vary depending on the size of the scallops.) Serve with bamboo toothpicks.

NOTES

You'll likely have leftover Bacon Jam. Refrigerate the jam for three to four days. It is great on crackers (such as part of the Charcuterie Board with Crackers and Artichoke Hummus on page 48) and can even be served on burgers!

COCONUT SHRIMP WITH PINEAPPLE DIPPING SAUCE

Seriously. You won't believe how easy it is to make this AIP-friendly recipe! Serve as an appetizer or even as a main dish with a side salad.

PREP TIME 20 minutes   **COOK TIME** 10 minutes   **YIELD** Makes 3 to 4 servings

FOR THE DIPPING SAUCE

½ cup (185 g) coconut-based yogurt

¼ cup (43 g) cubed pineapple

2 teaspoons coconut aminos

¼ teaspoon sea salt, plus more as needed

FOR THE SHRIMP

12 ounces (340 g) shrimp, peeled and deveined

¼ cup (36 g) arrowroot starch

½ cup (112 g) coconut oil, melted, divided, plus more as needed

1 cup (80 g) shredded unsweetened coconut

1 teaspoon garlic powder

½ teaspoon sea salt

1. To make the dipping sauce: In a blender, combine all the ingredients and lightly blend. Taste and adjust the seasoning, if desired. Set aside.

2. To make the shrimp: Set up a dipping station with the shrimp on a clean plate, the arrowroot starch in a bowl, ¼ cup (60 ml) of melted coconut oil in another bowl, the shredded coconut mixed with garlic powder and salt in a third bowl, and another clean plate to transfer the coated shrimp to.

3. Working one at a time, thoroughly coat the shrimp by dipping it into the arrowroot starch, then the coconut oil, then the coconut mixture, and finally transferring it to the clean plate.

4. In a large deep pan over medium-high heat, heat the remaining ¼ cup (56 g) of coconut oil.

5. Carefully add half the shrimp to the hot oil. Fry for about 2 minutes on each side or until the coating and shrimp are cooked. Using tongs or a slotted spoon, transfer to a clean serving dish. Repeat with the remaining shrimp. Serve with the dipping sauce on the side.

VEGGIE TOTS

Tater Tots are a classic kids' favorite. We're used to them coming frozen in a big bag or in a greasy container from a fast-food restaurant or school cafeteria. Regardless of where they come from, classic tots are typically anything but healthy. Not these! These tots are loaded with veggies but taste so delicious that kids still love them!

PREP TIME 20 minutes   **COOK TIME** 25 minutes   **YIELD** Makes 20 to 25 veggie tots

3 tablespoons (42 g) coconut oil, plus more for preparing the baking sheet

1 heaping cup (120 g) zucchini, chopped

1 heaping cup (71 g) broccoli florets

½ cup (55 g) shredded carrot

¼ cup plus 1 tablespoon (35 g) coconut flour

¼ cup (30 g) tapioca starch

2 tablespoons (12 g) sliced scallion

1 tablespoon (4 g) chopped fresh parsley

1 teaspoon onion powder

½ teaspoon sea salt

1 Gelatin Egg (page 26)

1. Preheat the oven to 400°F (200°C, or gas marker 6) and line a baking sheet with parchment paper. Lightly coat it with coconut oil and set aside.

2. In a food processor, combine the zucchini, broccoli, and carrot and process until finely chopped. Transfer the vegetables to a nut milk bag, cheesecloth, or paper towel and strain out the excess water. Place the vegetables in a large bowl and stir in the coconut flour, tapioca starch, scallion, parsley, onion powder, and salt.

3. Fold in the coconut oil.

4. Prepare the gelatin egg and immediately add it to the mixture. Mix well to combine. Form the vegetable mixture into small, 1-inch (2.5 cm) tots. (You should have 20 to 25.) Place them on the prepared baking sheet, spaced evenly. Bake for 25 minutes, carefully flipping with tongs halfway through the baking time.

5. Let cool. Serve with Nightshade-Free Ketchup (page 30), or enjoy alone.

Also pictured, Nightshade-Free Ketchup, page 30 →

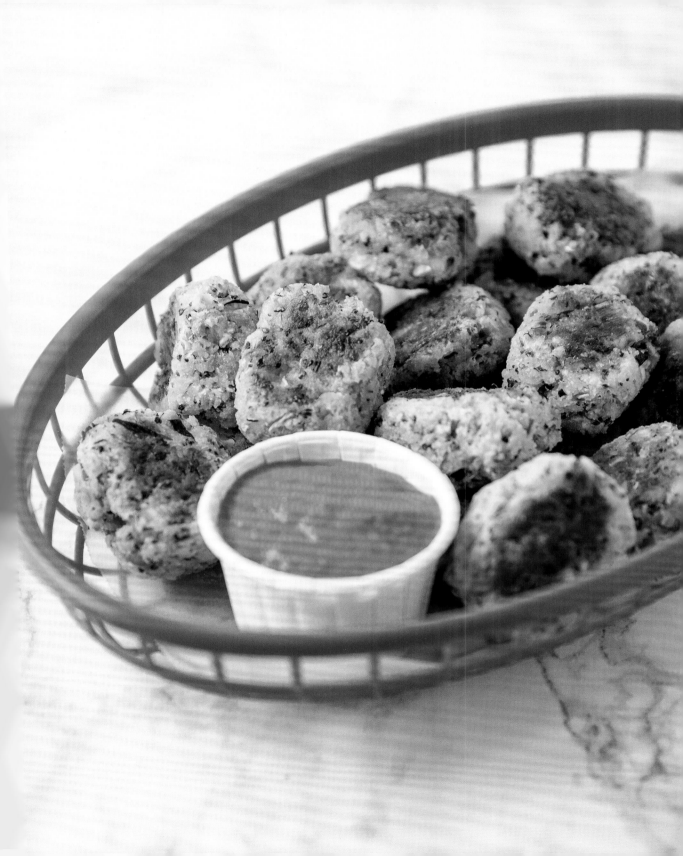

SALT AND VINEGAR CARROT CHIPS

My husband *loves* salt and vinegar chips, and I love to have this healthy, AIP-compliant option he can enjoy. Use large carrots with the biggest diameter for bigger chips.

PREP TIME 10 minutes   **COOK TIME** 20 minutes   **YIELD** Makes 2 servings

2 large carrots, peeled, ends trimmed

2 tablespoons (28 ml) avocado oil

1 tablespoon (15 ml) apple cider vinegar

1 teaspoon sea salt

1. Preheat the oven to 425°F (220°C, or gas mark 7) and line a baking sheet with parchment paper. Set aside.

2. Using a mandoline, carefully slice the carrots into ⅛-inch (3 mm)-thick slices. You should have about 2 cups (244 g) of carrot chips. Place the chips in a large bowl. Add the avocado oil, vinegar, and salt and toss until thoroughly coated. Lay the chips onto the prepared baking sheet, spaced evenly. Bake for 20 minutes, flipping halfway through the baking time. Carefully watch the chips for the last 5 minutes or so of cook time and remove any smaller chips baking more quickly than others.

3. Keep refrigerated and enjoy as a snack or appetizer.

PLANTAIN CHIPS

This sweet tropical fruit is the starchier cousin to the banana, but doesn't taste much like it. When you thinly slice it and bake it, you're in for a seriously good chip.

PREP TIME 10 minutes   **COOK TIME** 20 minutes   **YIELD** Makes 3 servings

2 green plantains, ends trimmed

2 tablespoons (28 ml) avocado oil

½ teaspoon sea salt

Juice of ½ lime

1. Preheat the oven to 375°F (190°C, or gas mark 5) and line a baking sheet with parchment paper. Set aside.

2. Make a slice in the center of the plantain peels and peel them back. Using a mandoline, carefully slice the plantains into ⅛-inch (3 mm)-thick slices. Lay the slices on the prepared baking sheet, spaced evenly, and coat with the avocado oil, salt, and lime juice. Bake for 15 to 20 minutes, rotating once or twice to cook evenly, or until crispy.

3. Serve with Queso Blanco (page 60), optional, or Guacamole (page 59), optional, for dipping.

GUACAMOLE

It's not a party without guacamole! You don't need nightshade spices to make this guacamole taste delicious. It still has bit of a kick from the garlic and red onion.

PREP TIME 10 minutes   **YIELD** Makes 4 servings

2 medium ripe avocados, halved, pitted, and flesh scooped out

2 tablespoons (28 ml) avocado oil

Juice of 1 lime

1 garlic clove, minced

½ red onion, diced

2 tablespoons (2 g) chopped fresh cilantro

½ teaspoon sea salt, plus more as needed

1. In a medium bowl, combine the avocado flesh, avocado oil, and lime juice. Using a fork, mash until smooth.

2. Stir in the garlic, red onion, cilantro, and salt. Taste, adjust the seasoning, and serve fresh.

NOTES

Guacamole will turn brown if left out for extended periods of time and is best eaten fresh. Extend the life by topping it with more lime juice to delay oxidation.

QUESO BLANCO

Get game day started on the right foot with this dairy-free "cheese" dip that will remind you of the familiar queso blanco, which means "white cheese" in Spanish. It is often made using melted American and Monterey Jack cheeses. Serve this version with Plantain Chips (page 59) or sliced vegetables.

PREP TIME 25 minutes   **COOK TIME** 10 minutes   **YIELD** Makes 5 to 6 servings

1 cup (200 g) cooked, mashed Hannah sweet potato (see Notes)

1 cup (235 ml) coconut milk

⅔ cup (160 ml) Chicken Bone Broth (page 25)

2 tablespoons (7.5 g) nutritional yeast

1 teaspoon onion powder

1 teaspoon garlic powder

½ teaspoon sea salt

1 tablespoon (9 g) arrowroot starch

1 teaspoon apple cider vinegar

1 tablespoon (1 g) chopped fresh cilantro

Plantain Chips (page 59), for serving

1. In a high-speed blender or food processor, combine the mashed sweet potato, coconut milk, bone broth, nutritional yeast, onion powder, garlic powder, and salt. Blend until smooth and transfer to a saucepan over medium heat.

2. Whisk in the arrowroot starch. Cook for 5 minutes, stirring constantly to thicken the mixture.

3. Whisk in the vinegar. Remove from the pan from the heat and divide the mixture among five or six bowls. Top with the cilantro and serve with the Plantain Chips.

Also pictured, Plantain Chips, page 59 →

NOTES

Hannah sweet potatoes are the best variety for this queso as they are the least sweet. If you can't find them, use another white-fleshed sweet potato.

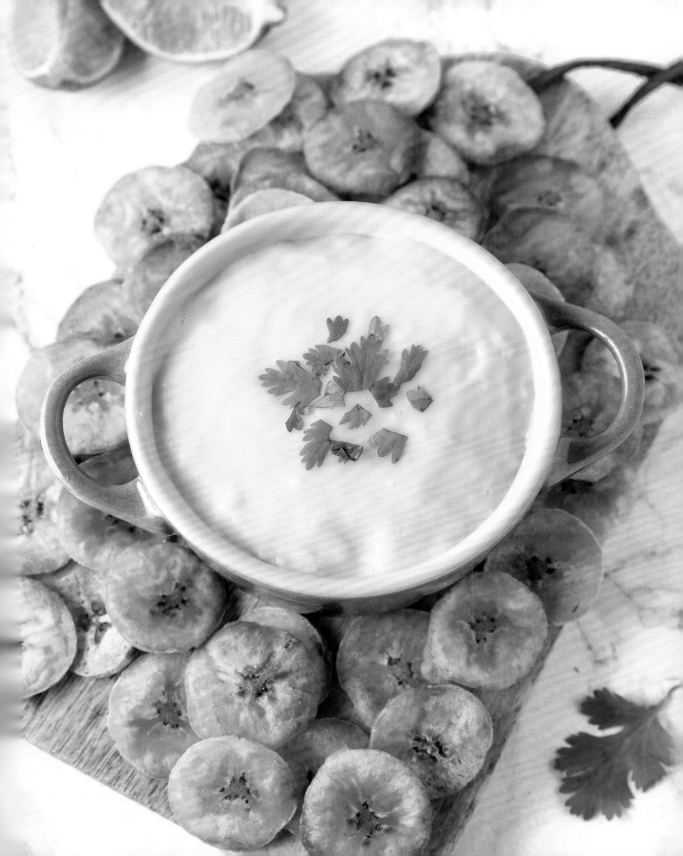

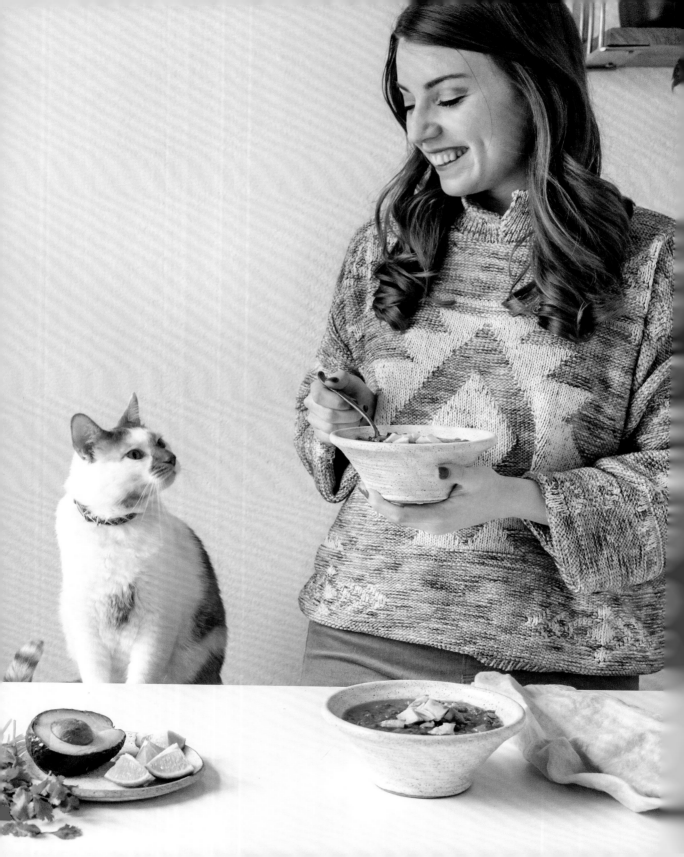

CHAPTER 5

SOUPS, SALADS & SIDES

Soups can be an incredibly healing and nourishing staple to have on the AIP, and salads and vegetable-rich side dishes add extra nutrients, textures, and flavors to a meal. Having the right soup or salad to start a meal or a good side dish to pair with a protein can immediately elevate and round out what could be an otherwise boring meal. I don't know how I would get through winter without a warming soup such as Butternut Bison Chili (page 77), or summer without a light, crisp dish such as Picnic Broccoli Slaw (page 88)!

← Butternut Bison Chili, page 77

BROCCOLI "CHEESE" SOUP

This creamy, cheesy soup is the perfect way to get some extra broccoli into your diet! Nutritional yeast and coconut milk are the substitutes for cheese and cream in this AIP take on a classic.

PREP TIME 10 minutes   **COOK TIME** 35 minutes   **YIELD** Makes 4 servings

2 tablespoons (28 g) coconut oil

½ medium onion, diced

4 cups (284 g) bite-size broccoli florets

1 cup (110 g) shredded carrot

2 cups (475 ml) Chicken Bone Broth (page 25)

2 cups (475 ml) coconut milk

⅓ cup (80 g) coconut cream

3 tablespoons (11.5 g) nutritional yeast

½ teaspoon sea salt, plus more as needed

2 teaspoons arrowroot starch

1. In a large pot over medium heat, melt the coconut oil.

2. Add the onion and sauté for 5 to 6 minutes or until translucent.

3. Add the broccoli, carrot, bone broth, coconut milk, coconut cream, nutritional yeast, and salt and stir well to combine. Bring to a simmer and cook for 20 to 25 minutes or until the vegetables are fork-tender.

4. Stir in the arrowroot starch and simmer for 1 minute more to thicken the soup slightly. Taste, adjust the seasoning, and serve warm.

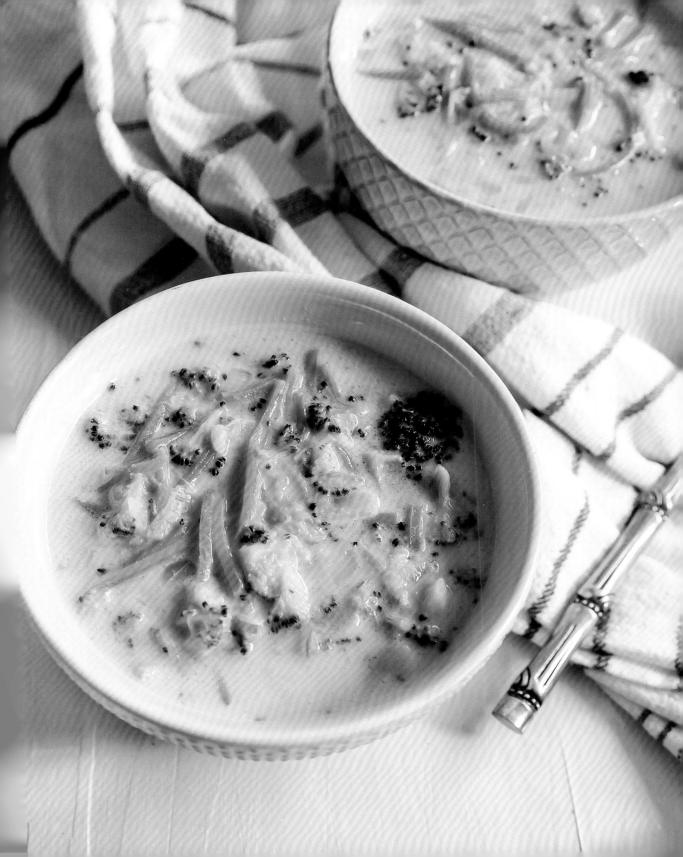

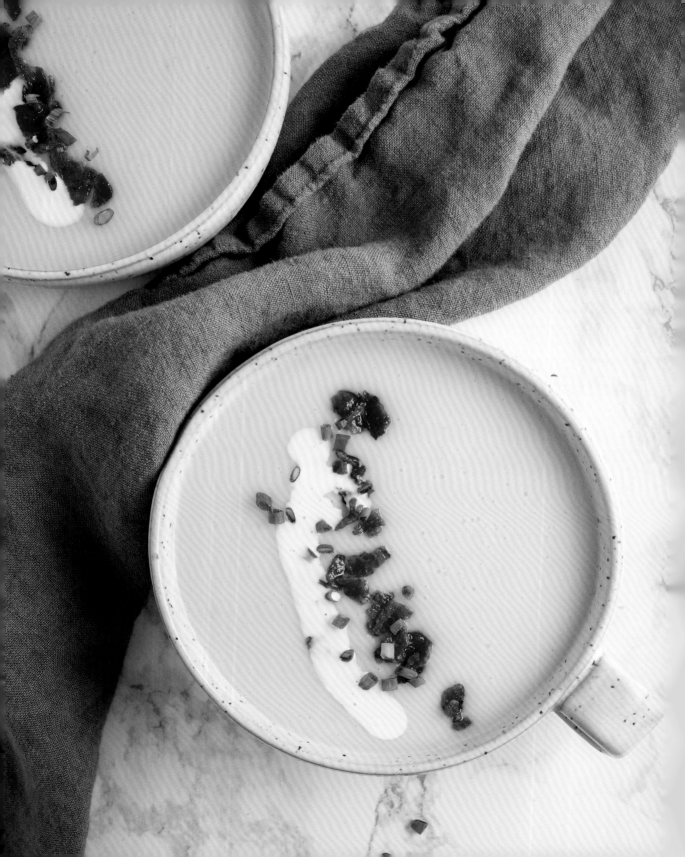

CHAPTER 6

CRAVEABLE MAINS & PROTEINS

It can be easy to become bored when following a diet, but it also becomes more challenging when you're omitting a wide variety of foods. Getting stuck in a food rut is common, but there is so much more to nourishing AIP meals than just chicken, broccoli, and sweet potato. This chapter features the special Sunday night dinner you've been looking for, the easy one-pan meal you need for a weeknight, and more!

← Sloppy Joe Casserole, page 110

STEAK & FRIES

Serve this meal for date night, on Valentine's Day, at anniversaries, or simply for an extra-special Sunday night! The sweet potato fries pair well with other meals as a simple side.

PREP TIME 20 minutes   **COOK TIME** 40 minutes   **YIELD** Makes 2 servings

FOR THE SWEET POTATO FRIES

1 large sweet potato, or 2 medium, scrubbed well and cut into thin fries

2 tablespoons (28 ml) avocado oil

½ teaspoon sea salt

1 teaspoon garlic powder

Nightshade-Free Ketchup, for serving (optional)

FOR THE STEAK

2 rib eye steaks (1 to 1½ pounds [455 to 680 g] total)

1 teaspoon sea salt

2 tablespoons (28 ml) avocado oil

4 thyme sprigs

2 rosemary sprigs

2 garlic cloves, peeled

1. To make the sweet potato fries: Preheat the oven to 400°F (200°C, or gas mark 6) and line a baking sheet with parchment paper.

2. Place the fries on the prepared baking sheet, add the avocado oil, and toss to coat. Sprinkle with the salt and garlic powder. Bake for 35 to 40 minutes, flipping halfway through the baking time, until the fries reach your desired crispness.

3. Set aside to cool slightly before serving with the ketchup (if using).

4. To make the steak: While the fries cook, pat the steaks dry and season both sides with salt. Let sit on the counter for 15 minutes.

5. In a cast iron skillet over medium-high heat, heat the avocado oil.

6. Once the oil is hot, carefully add the steaks to the skillet, along with the thyme, rosemary, and garlic. Cook for 3 minutes on each side until seared. Continue to cook for 1 to 2 minutes more on each side, flipping every minute until the steaks reach your desired doneness (see Notes). Remove the steaks from the pan and discard the herb sprigs and garlic.

7. Let the steaks rest for 5 to 10 minutes before serving with the fries and a side such as Caesar Salad (page 83).

NOTES

Use a meat thermometer to check for doneness: 120°F to 125°F (49°C to 52°C) is rare; 130°F to 135°F (54°C to 57°C) is medium-rare; 140°F to 145°F (60°C to 63°C) is medium; 150°F to 155°F (66°C to 68°C) is medium-well, and beyond is well done.

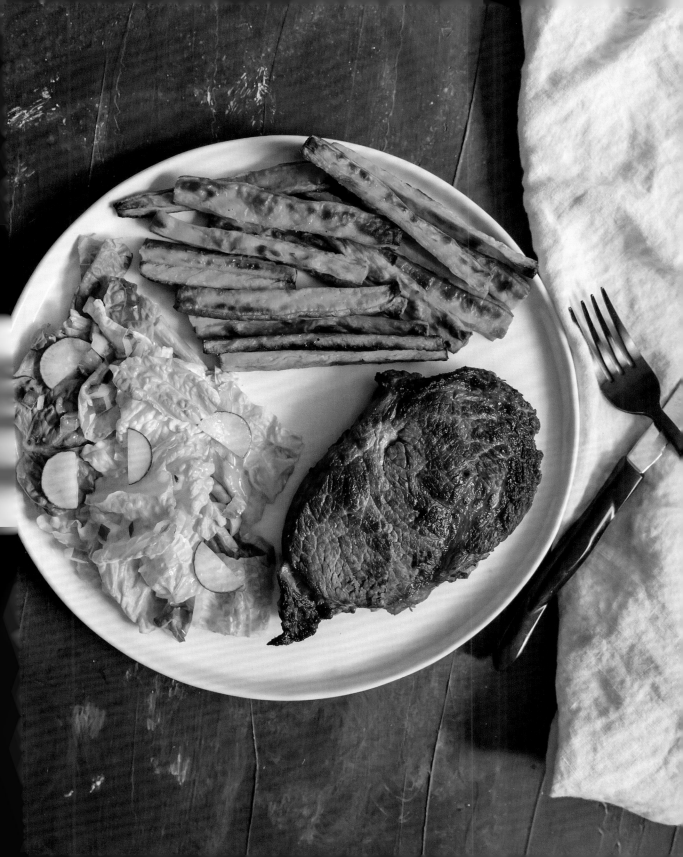

ITALIAN-STYLE MEATLOAF MUFFINS

Nothing says "comfort food" quite like meatloaf! It's nourishing, nostalgic, and simple to make. These meatloaf muffins are a twist on the classic that are fun to eat!

PREP TIME 10 minutes   **COOK TIME** 55 minutes   **YIELD** Makes 8 to 9 servings

1 tablespoon (15 ml) avocado oil

1 medium white onion, diced

2 garlic cloves, minced

1 pound (455 g) ground beef

1 pound (455 g) ground pork

1 tablespoon (3 g) chopped fresh basil leaves, plus more for garnishing

1 tablespoon (4 g) chopped fresh parsley

¾ to 1 teaspoon sea salt

1 cup (250 g) Nightshade-Free "Tomato" Sauce (page 31), warmed

1. Preheat the oven to 400°F (200°C, or gas mark 6).

2. In a medium skillet over low heat, heat the avocado oil.

3. Add the onion and garlic and sauté for 5 to 6 minutes or until the onion is translucent. Set aside.

4. In a large bowl, mix together the ground beef, ground pork, basil, parsley, and salt. Fold in the onion and garlic mixture and thoroughly combine. Evenly divide the mixture among 8 or 9 cups of a 12-cup muffin tin. Bake for 40 to 50 minutes or until the internal temperature reaches 160°F (71°C) on a meat thermometer.

5. Let cool slightly before topping with the "tomato" sauce and garnishing with basil.

NOTES

To make meal prep ready, store the meatloaf muffins and sauce separately. Reserve additional basil for garnish and store in glass containers for 3-4 days. Reheat the meatloaf muffins under the broiler, the sauce in a pot over medium heat, and add garnish to serve.

SLOW COOKER BARBECUE BRISKET

As a native New Yorker, I was skeptical about barbecue until I moved to Texas, where it's a delicious way of life. Serve this brisket with Sweet Potato Fries (page 96), Southern Fried Cabbage (page 83), or Picnic Broccoli Slaw (page 88).

PREP TIME 20 minutes **COOK TIME** 8 hours, 30 minutes **YIELD** Makes 8 servings

FOR THE BARBECUE SAUCE

1 tablespoon (15 ml) bacon fat, or avocado oil

1 medium white onion, diced

2 garlic cloves, minced

1 cup (130 g) chopped carrot

¼ cup (60 ml) water

2 tablespoons (40 g) blackstrap molasses

2 tablespoons (28 ml) apple cider vinegar

1 teaspoon coconut aminos

½ teaspoon smoked salt, plus more as needed

⅓ cup (52 g) dark pitted cherries

FOR THE BRISKET

3 pounds (1.46 kg) beef brisket

1 teaspoon smoked salt

2 tablespoons (28 ml) avocado oil

1 cup (235 ml) Beef Bone Broth (page 24)

1½ cups (375 g) Barbecue Sauce (recipe follows), divided

2 bay leaves

½ white onion, sliced

1. To make the barbecue sauce: In a medium saucepan over medium heat, heat the bacon fat.

2. Add the onion and garlic and sauté for 5 to 6 minutes, or until the onion is translucent.

3. Add the carrot and sauté for 5 minutes more until slightly softened.

4. Add the water, molasses, vinegar, coconut aminos, salt, and cherries and stir well to combine. Bring the mixture to a low simmer and cook for 10 minutes, stirring often, to thicken the sauce.

5. Let cool slightly before transferring to a high-speed blender and blending until smooth. Taste and adjust the seasoning.

6. To make the brisket: Season the brisket on both sides with salt.

7. In a large skillet over medium heat, heat the avocado oil.

8. Add the brisket and lightly sear on both sides. Drain the excess fat and add the brisket to a slow cooker.

9. Top the brisket with the bone broth and ¾ cup (188 g) of barbecue sauce, spreading the sauce evenly over the top of the brisket. Add the bay leaves and onion. Cover the slow cooker, set it to low, and cook for 8 hours.

10. Remove and discard the bay leaves and excess onions and remove the brisket. Use two forks to shred the brisket or slice it with a knife. Top with the remaining ¾ cup (188 g) of sauce and serve.

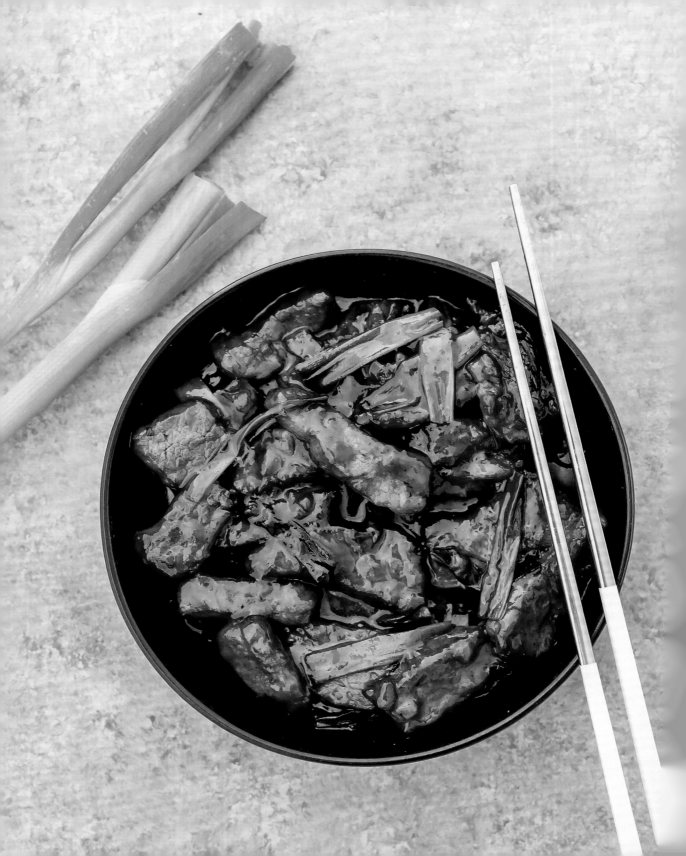

MONGOLIAN BEEF

You seriously won't believe this Mongolian beef is AIP compliant! This dish is so flavorful and rich it's sure to fool any guests—if you choose to share, that is!

PREP TIME 15 minutes **COOK TIME** 20 minutes **YIELD** Makes 3 to 4 servings

1 pound (455 g) flank steak

1 teaspoon sea salt, divided

1 tablespoon (9 g) arrowroot starch

2 tablespoons (28 ml) avocado oil

4 garlic cloves, minced

1-inch (2.5 cm) piece fresh ginger, peeled and grated

⅓ cup (80 ml) coconut aminos

¼ cup (60 ml) Beef Bone Broth (page 24), or water

4 scallions, chopped

1. Season the flank steak on both sides with salt. Using a sharp butcher's knife, slice the steak against the grain into thin 1-inch (2.5 cm)-long slices. Place the arrowroot starch in a shallow bowl and coat the steak slices in it.

2. In a large deep pan over medium heat, heat the avocado oil.

3. Once the oil is hot, carefully add half the beef and cook for 1 to 2 minutes on each side. The beef should be slightly crispy. Remove from the pan and set aside. Repeat with the remaining beef.

4. Add the garlic and ginger to the pan and cook for 2 to 3 minutes, or until fragrant.

5. Slightly reduce the heat and stir in the coconut aminos and bone broth. Return the beef to the pan and simmer for 3 to 5 minutes, stirring often. The sauce should thicken.

6. Add the scallions and cook for 1 minute more.

7. Remove the beef mixture from the pan and serve over Basic Cauliflower Rice (page 28) or the vegetables prepared in the Teriyaki Chicken Stir-Fry (page 135).

NOTES

To make this meal-prep ready, refrigerate this dish in individual glass containers for two to three days.

SWEDISH MEATBALLS

Swedish meatballs are creamy, savory and a perfect dish to serve when you want some variety in your dinner rotation. They are tasty with root vegetable mashes, such as sweet potato or Roasted Parsnip Mash (page 163).

PREP TIME 10 minutes   **COOK TIME** 35 minutes   **YIELD** Makes 13-15 meatballs

FOR THE MEATBALLS

1 pound (455 g) ground beef

½ white onion, finely diced

1 tablespoon (7 g) coconut flour

1 teaspoon salt

½ teaspoon ground mace

1 tablespoon (13 g) beef tallow

FOR THE SAUCE

1 cup (240 g) coconut cream

¾ cup (175 ml) Beef Bone Broth (page 25)

1 tablespoon (15 ml) coconut aminos

2 tablespoons (26 g) beef tallow

½ teaspoon sea salt

1 tablespoon (9 g) arrowroot starch

2 tablespoons (8 g) chopped fresh parsley

1. To make the meatballs: In a large bowl, mix together the ground beef, onion, coconut flour, salt, and mace until well combined. Roll the mixture into 12 meatballs and set aside.

2. In a large skillet over medium heat, heat the beef tallow.

3. Add the meatballs to the skillet and fry for 7 to 10 minutes until browned and cooked through. Transfer to a plate. Discard the fat from the pan and remove any browned bits.

4. To make the sauce: Return the skillet to medium heat and add the coconut cream, bone broth, coconut aminos, beef tallow, and salt. Stir well. Bring to a simmer and cook for 5 minutes.

5. Whisk in the arrowroot starch and let the sauce thicken.

6. Add the meatballs to the skillet and reheat for 2 to 3 minutes, coating the meatballs in the sauce. Top with the parsley. Serve alone over a vegetable mash of choice.

NOTES

To make meal-prep ready, reserve garnish and store in glass for 3-4 days. Reheat in a pan over medium heat, and add garnish.

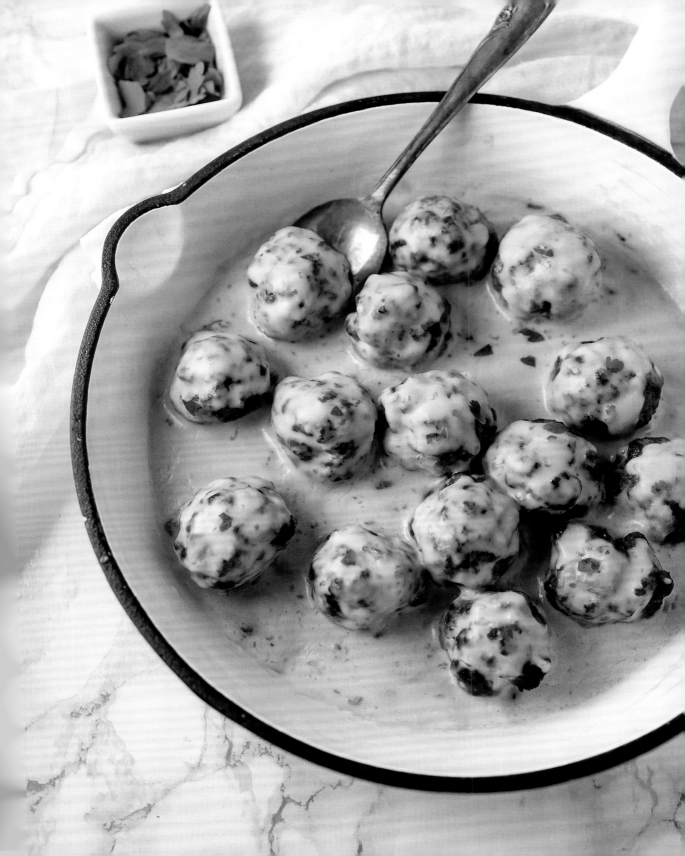

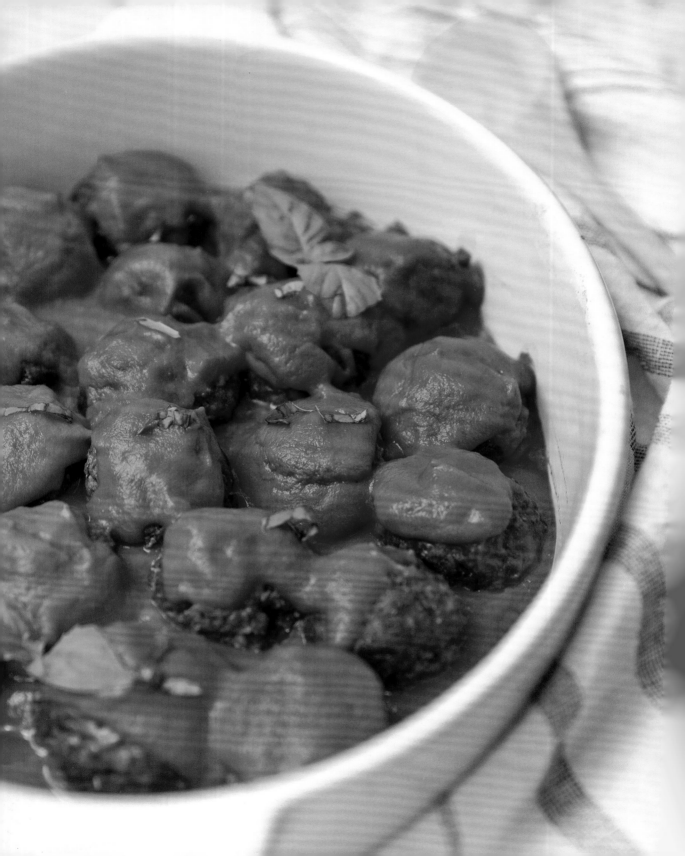

ITALIAN-STYLE MEATBALLS

Traditionally, meatballs are made with eggs and bread crumbs to bind them. Can you really get by without these ingredients? Yes, you can! These AIP-friendly meatballs taste just as delicious as those that my Italian-American family was famous for making.

PREP TIME 15 minutes   **COOK TIME** 25 minutes
YIELD Makes 20 to 22 meatballs

1 pound (455 g) ground beef

1 small onion, finely diced

2 garlic cloves, finely minced

1 tablespoon (3 g) chopped fresh basil leaves, divided

2 teaspoons chopped fresh parsley

1 teaspoon dried oregano

½ teaspoon sea salt

2 to 3 cups (500 to 750 g) Nightshade-Free "Tomato" Sauce (page 31), warmed

1. Preheat the oven to 400°F (200°C, or gas mark 6) and line a baking sheet with parchment paper. Set aside.

2. In a medium bowl, combine the ground beef, onion, garlic, half the basil (reserving the other half for garnishing), the parsley, oregano, and salt until fully incorporated. Roll the mixture into 1½-inch (3.5 cm) meatballs. You should have 20 to 22 meatballs. Place them on the prepared baking sheet and bake for 20 to 25 minutes, or until fully cooked.

3. Serve with the warm "tomato" sauce and garnish with the reserved basil.

NOTES

To make this meal-prep ready, refrigerate in individual glass storage containers and eat for lunches with a side dish, such as Zucchini Noodles (see Bolognese with Zucchini Noodles, page 109) or a salad, throughout the week.

ZUCCHINI LASAGNA

Lasagna is my family's love language. My mom was constantly cooking lasagna, and my husband is just as big of a fan! Lasagna traditionally contains at least three different cheeses so it was a feat adapting this classic to be AIP compliant.

PREP TIME 30 minutes   **COOK TIME** 45 minutes   **YIELD** Makes 6 servings

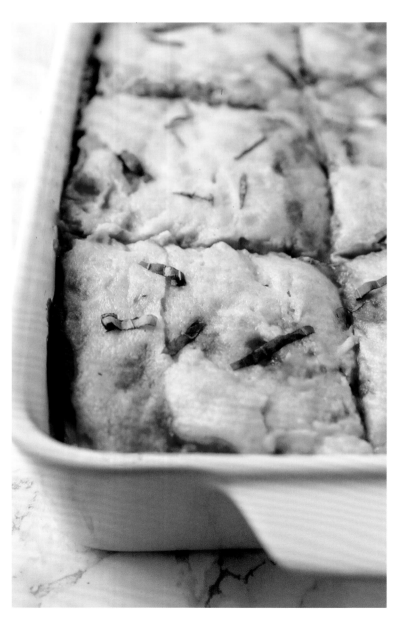

FOR THE CAULIFLOWER "CHEESE"

1½ cups (150 g) cauliflower, steamed

1 teaspoon lemon juice

2 tablespoons (28 ml) olive oil

1 tablespoon (7 g) gelatin

2 tablespoons (7.5 g nutritional yeast

1 tablespoon (7.5 g) tapioca starch

¼ teaspoon sea salt

FOR THE LASAGNA

1 tablespoon (15 ml) olive oil

2 garlic cloves, minced

1 medium onion, diced

2 cups (140 g) sliced mushrooms

2 cups (60 g) fresh spinach, chopped

1 pound (454 g) ground beef

¾ teaspoon sea salt (plus further to taste)

1¼ cups (312.5 g) Nightshade-Free "Tomato" Sauce (page 31), divided

4 large zucchini, ends trimmed

2 tablespoons (6 g) chopped fresh basil leaves

1. Line a large baking sheet with parchment paper and set aside.

2. To make the cauliflower "cheese:" While the cauliflower is still warm use a nut milk bag, cheesecloth, or paper towel to lightly strain some, but not all, excess water from the steamed cauliflower. Transfer to a food processor.

3. Add the remaining "cheese" ingredients and blend until smooth. Pour onto the prepared baking sheet and spread into a thin, even layer. Freeze for 10 to 15 minutes or until set.

4. To make the lasagna: In a large skillet over low heat, heat the olive oil.

5. Add the garlic and onion and sauté for 5 to 6 minutes or until the onion is translucent.

6. Add the mushrooms and sauté for 4 to 5 minutes or until soft.

7. Add the spinach, stirring until it wilts. Remove the vegetables from the skillet and set aside. Wipe the oil from the pan.

8. Return the skillet to medium heat and add the ground beef and salt. Sauté for 7 to 10 minutes or until browned, breaking it up with the back of a spoon.

9. Stir in the vegetable mixture and ½ cup (125 g) of the "tomato" sauce. Set aside.

10. Using a vegetable peeler or mandoline set to ⅛ inch (3 mm), cut long, thin "sheets" from the zucchini. Set aside for 5 minutes and pat dry with a paper towel or clean dishtowel.

11. Preheat the oven to 375°F (190°C, or gas mark 5).

12. Coat the bottom of a 9 x 13-inch (23 x 33 cm) baking pan with ¼ cup (63 g) of "tomato" sauce. Cover the bottom of the pan with one layer of zucchini sheets. Top with the beef and vegetable mixture. Repeat the layering one more time.

13. Top the lasagna with a final layer of zucchini, ½ cup (125 g) of the "tomato" sauce, and the "cheese." If necessary, break up the cauliflower "cheese" to cover the lasagna fully. Bake for 15 to 20 minutes or until the "cheese" has melted and the zucchini sheets are soft. Serve topped with the basil.

SWEET POTATO SHEPHERD'S PIE

Shepherd's pie is classic comfort food that conveniently makes a full, nourishing meal. This dish is traditionally made with white potatoes, but it tastes just as delicious with sweet potato.

PREP TIME 10 minutes   **COOK TIME** 20 minutes   **YIELD** Makes 4 servings

5 cups (665 g) peeled chopped sweet potato

2 tablespoons (28 g) coconut oil, divided

1 teaspoon sea salt, divided

1 medium onion, diced

1 cup (130 g) diced carrot

1 pound (455 g) ground beef

¼ cup (62.5 g) Nightshade-Free "Tomato" Sauce (page 31)

¼ cup (60 ml) Beef Bone Broth (page 24)

2 teaspoons coconut aminos

2 teaspoons fresh rosemary leaves, chopped

1 teaspoon fresh thyme leaves, chopped

2 teaspoons chopped fresh parsley

1. In a large pot, combine the sweet potato and enough water to cover. Place the pot over medium-high heat and bring to a simmer. Cook until the potatoes are fork-tender. Strain and let cool slightly. Transfer to a food processor. Add 1 tablespoon (14 g) of coconut oil and a pinch of salt and blend until smooth. Set aside.

2. In a large skillet over medium heat, melt the remaining 1 tablespoon (14 g) of coconut oil.

3. Add the onion and sauté for 5 to 6 minutes or until translucent.

4. Add the carrot and sauté for 5 to 7 minutes or just until fork-tender.

5. Add the ground beef and salt. Cook for 7 to 10 minutes or until the beef is browned, breaking it up with the back of a spoon.

6. Stir in the "tomato" sauce, bone broth, coconut aminos, and herbs. Cook for 5 to 10 minutes to thicken.

7. Preheat the oven to 400°F (200°C, or gas mark 6).

8. Spoon the beef and vegetable mixture into a 9 x 13-inch (22 x 23 cm) baking dish. Spread the mashed sweet potato on top. Use a fork or spoon to create soft peaks in the potatoes or add decorative lines. Bake for 25 to 30 minutes and serve.

BOLOGNESE WITH ZUCCHINI NOODLES

Take Italian night to the next level with this rich and hearty Bolognese sauce served with zoodles for the full pasta experience!

PREP TIME 20 minutes **COOK TIME** 55 minutes **YIELD** Makes 4 servings

**FOR THE
BOLOGNESE SAUCE**

1 pound (455 g) ground beef

½ teaspoon sea salt, divided, plus more as needed

2 tablespoons (28 ml) olive oil

1 medium onion, diced

2 garlic cloves, chopped

½ cup (65 g) finely diced carrot

½ cup (60 g) finely chopped celery

1½ cups (375 g) Nightshade-Free "Tomato" Sauce (page 31)

1 cup (235 ml) Chicken Bone Broth (page 25)

2 teaspoons dried oregano

1 tablespoon (3 g) chopped fresh basil leaves

1 tablespoon (4 g) chopped fresh parsley

FOR THE ZOODLES

4 large zucchini, ends trimmed, spiralized

1 teaspoon salt

2 teaspoons olive oil

1. To make the bolognese sauce: In a large deep skillet with a lid over medium heat, combine the ground beef and ¼ teaspoon of salt. Brown the beef for 7 to 10 minutes, breaking it up with the back of spoon. Using a slotted spoon, remove the beef and drain the majority of fat from the skillet.

2. Return the skillet to medium-low heat and add the olive oil to heat.

3. Add the onion and garlic and sauté for 5 to 6 minutes, or until the onion is translucent.

4. Stir in the carrot and celery and cook for 3 to 4 minutes more.

5. Add the cooked beef, "tomato" sauce, bone broth, remaining ¼ teaspoon of salt, and oregano. Stir well to combine. Bring to a low simmer and cover the skillet. Cook for about 30 minutes, or until the mixture is thickened and the vegetables are fork-tender.

6. Stir in the basil and parsley, taste, adjust the seasoning, and keep warm while you make the zoodles.

7. To make the zoodles: Put the zucchini noodles in a large bowl and sprinkle with the salt. Let sit for about 5 minutes to draw out the moisture. Use a paper towel to remove some of the liquid from the noodles.

8. In another skillet over low heat, heat the olive oil.

9. Add the zucchini noodles and sauté for 2 minutes or until just barely cooked. Serve topped with the Bolognese Sauce.

SLOPPY JOE CASSEROLE

I remember these classic sandwiches of ground beef in a sugary sauce served between two white buns in my school cafeteria and for dinner at friends' houses. Admit it—In some weird way, they tasted pretty good. This sloppy joe casserole tastes like a real-food version of the classic recipe topped with crispy sweet potato tots.

PREP TIME 30 minutes   **COOK TIME** 1 hour   **YIELD** Makes 5 to 6 servings

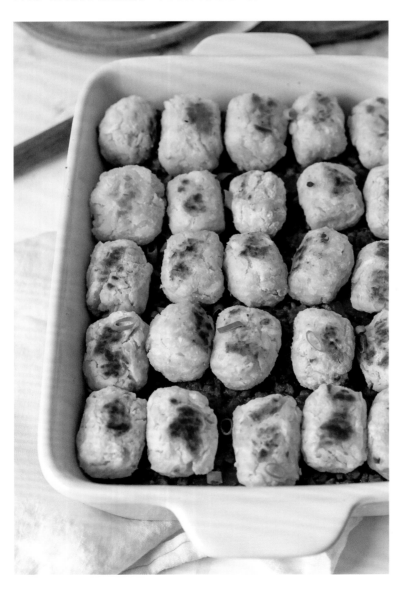

FOR THE SWEET POTATO TOTS

2 medium white or orange sweet potatoes, peeled

2 tablespoons (14 g) coconut flour

2 teaspoons garlic powder

2 teaspoons onion powder

1 teaspoon sea salt

2 tablespoons (28 ml) avocado oil

FOR THE SAUCE

1 cup (333 g) Nightshade-Free Ketchup (page 30)

½ cup (120 ml) water

1 tablespoon (15 ml) coconut aminos

2 teaspoons coconut sugar

1 teaspoon apple cider vinegar

1 teaspoon garlic powder

½ teaspoon sea salt

FOR THE SLOPPY JOES

2 tablespoons (28 g) coconut oil, or (28 ml) avocado oil, divided

1 pound (455 g) ground beef

1 medium onion, finely diced

2 scallions, chopped

1. To make the sweet potato tots: Bring a large pot of water to a low boil over medium heat and add the whole sweet potatoes. Use a wooden spoon to keep them mostly submerged. Cook for 20 minutes. Remove from the water and set aside to cool.

2. Meanwhile, preheat the oven to 400°F (200°C, or gas mark 6) and line a baking sheet with parchment paper. Set aside.

3. Using a box grater, grate the sweet potatoes. Squeeze out the excess water with a paper towel or cheesecloth. Place in a medium bowl.

4. Stir in the coconut flour, garlic powder, onion powder, salt, and 1 tablespoon (15 ml) of avocado oil. Form the sweet potato mixture into 1-inch (2.5 cm) tots (you should have about 25) and place them on the prepared baking sheet, spaced evenly. Drizzle with the remaining 1 tablespoon (15 ml) of avocado oil. Bake for 20 to 25 minutes, carefully flipping them halfway through the baking time.

5. Remove and set aside when done, leaving the oven on.

6. To make the sauce: In a large bowl, whisk all the sauce ingredients until combined. Set aside.

7. To make the sloppy joe casserole: While the sweet potato tots are cooking, in a large skillet over medium heat, melt 1 tablespoon (14 g) of coconut oil.

8. Add the ground beef and onion to the skillet. Cook for about 7 minutes, breaking up the meat with a wooden spoon or spatula, until the meat is browned. Remove from the heat and drain most of the fat from the skillet. Return the skillet to medium heat.

9. Stir in the sauce. Bring to a simmer and cook for 8 to 10 minutes. Transfer the mixture to a 9 x 6-inch (23 x 15 cm) casserole dish.

10. Place the sweet potato tots on top of the Sloppy Joe mixture in an evenly spaced pattern. Bake for 6 to 8 minutes or until the casserole is warm. Top with the scallions and serve.

SLOW COOKER POT ROAST

Pot roast is filling, warming, and the all-around perfect slow cooker meal. Although this is one of those recipes I make on repeat during the winter, I never get tired of it.

PREP TIME 10 minutes   **COOK TIME** 8 hours   **YIELD** Makes 2 to 3 servings

3 to 4 pounds (1.4 to 1.8 kg) beef chuck roast

1 to 1½ teaspoons sea salt, plus more as needed

2 tablespoons (28 ml) avocado oil

2 cups (260 g) chopped carrot

1 medium onion, quartered

3 rosemary sprigs

3 thyme sprigs

2 bay leaves

1 cup (235 ml) Beef Bone Broth (page 24)

1. Season both sides of the roast with salt. In a large skillet over medium heat, heat the avocado oil.

2. Add the roast and gently sear for about 1 minute on each side. Carefully transfer the chuck roast into a slow cooker.

3. Add the carrot, onion, rosemary, thyme, and bay leaves. Pour in the bone broth. Cover the slow cooker, set it to low, and cook for 8 hours.

4. Remove and discard the bay leaves and serve warm.

NOTES

To make this meal-prep ready, portion the roast and vegetables into individual glass containers and refrigerate to have ready to enjoy throughout the week.

SLOW COOKER CARNITAS

I never had carnitas before I moved to Texas—and, boy, was I missing out! Carnitas are perfect for making nachos, burrito bowls, or just eating by themselves with a vegetable side dish. This recipe is flavorful and simple.

PREP TIME 15 minutes   **COOK TIME** 8 hours   **YIELD** Makes 8 servings

3 garlic cloves, minced

2 teaspoons dried cilantro

2 teaspoons dried oregano

1 teaspoon ground cinnamon

1 teaspoon sea salt

3 pounds (1.4 kg) pork shoulder

2 bay leaves

2 medium onions, quartered

1 cup (235 ml) fresh orange juice

Juice of 2 limes

1 to 2 tablespoons (1 to 2 g) fresh cilantro

1 to 2 limes, sliced

1. In a small bowl, stir together the garlic, cilantro, oregano, cinnamon, and salt. Evenly coat the pork on all sides with the spice rub and place it into a slow cooker.

2. Top the pork with the bay leaves, onion, and orange and lime juices. Cover the slow cooker, set it to low, and cook for 8 hours.

3. Remove the pork from the slow cooker and shred it with two forks. Top with the cilantro and serve with the limes.

4. If you like a crispier bite, place the carnitas on a large baking sheet and broil for 3 to 5 minutes or until slightly crisp.

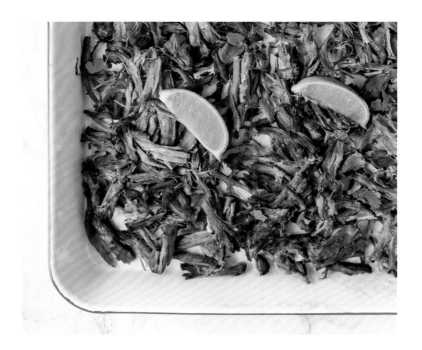

NOTES

Make this recipe into nachos by serving it with Plantain Chips (page 59) and Guacamole (page 59), or burrito bowls with Basic Cauliflower Rice (page 28), lettuce, and avocado.

ONE-PAN BEEF FAJITAS

Sheet pan fajitas are a fun, easy dish, but typically nightshade heavy. I come from a family of fajita lovers, and I would ask my mom to wait until I left the house to make them whenever I came home from college because the smell gave me headaches! You don't have to worry about noncompliant ingredients in this simple, delicious recipe.

PREP TIME 20 minutes   **COOK TIME** 20 minutes   **YIELD** Makes 4 servings

1 pound (455 g) flank steak, or skirt steak, cut against the grain into long thin slices

1 teaspoon sea salt, divided

3 tablespoons (45 ml) avocado oil

Juice of ½ lime

3 garlic cloves, minced

2 teaspoons dried oregano

2 zucchini, ends trimmed, cut into long thin strips

2 yellow squashes, ends trimmed, cut into long thin strips

1 medium red onion, halved, cut into thin half-moons

2 cups (140 g) mushrooms, sliced

3 tablespoons (3 g) chopped fresh cilantro

2 or 3 limes, quartered

1. Preheat the oven to 400°F (200°C, or gas mark 6) and line a large baking sheet with parchment paper. Set aside.

2. Season the steak with ½ teaspoon of salt and set aside in a large bowl.

3. In another large bowl, whisk the avocado oil, lime juice, garlic, oregano, and the remaining ½ teaspoon of salt.

4. Add the zucchini, squash, red onion, mushrooms, and steak to the marinade and toss to coat.

5. Transfer to the prepared baking sheet and cook for 20 to 22 minutes or until the vegetables and steak reached their desired doneness.

6. Transfer to plates, top with the cilantro, and serve with the lime wedges.

NOTES

Allow the uncooked steak to rest on the counter top for 15 minutes to allow to come to room temperature.

To make this meal-prep ready, refrigerate in individual glass containers for two to three days. Refer to Steak & Fries (page 96) for steak temperatures.

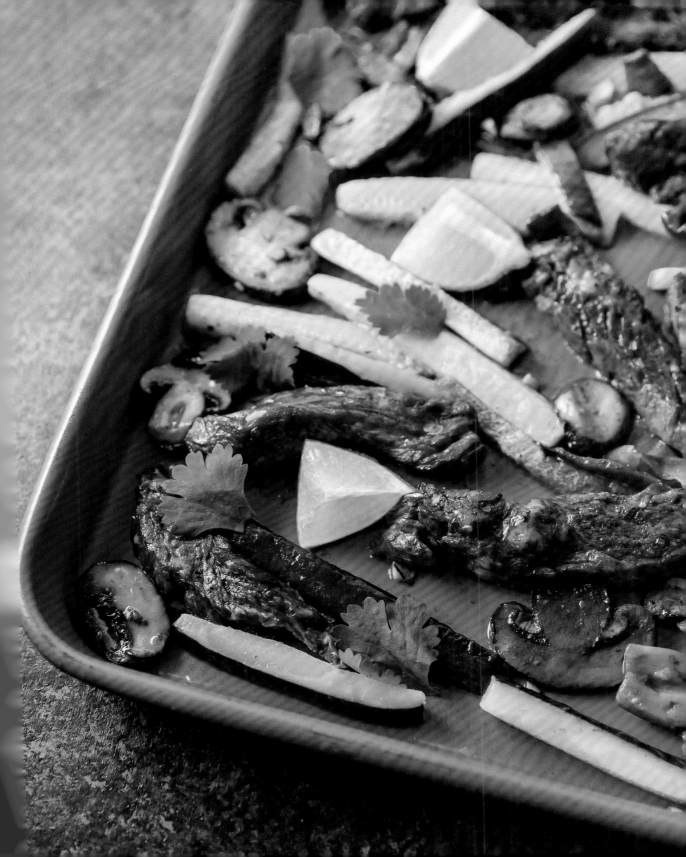

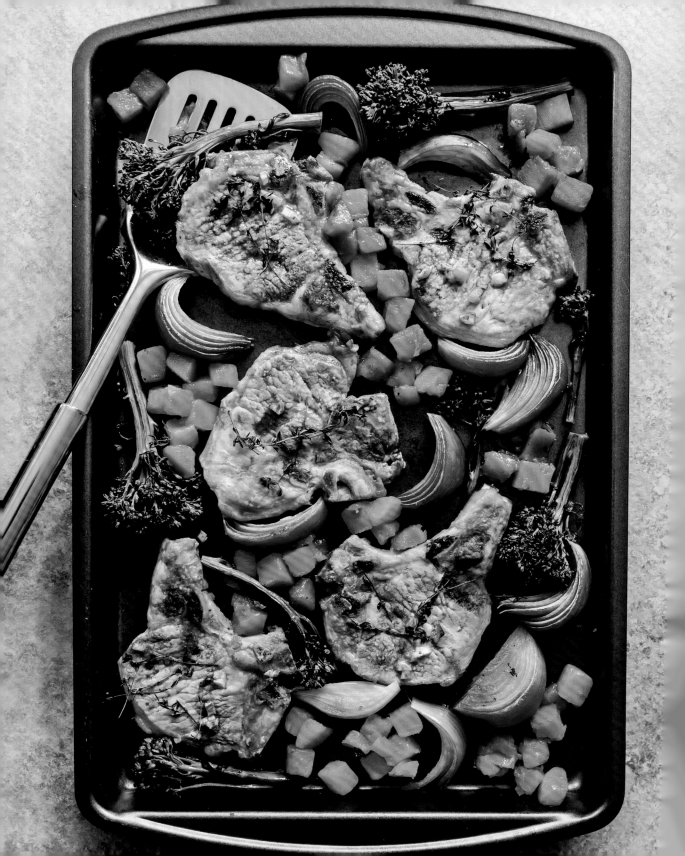

BALSAMIC PORK CHOP DINNER

Crunched for time on a Tuesday night but still want something hearty and filling? This simple one-pan meal has you covered in just about 45 minutes!

PREP TIME 15 minutes   **COOK TIME** 30 minutes
YIELD Makes 4 to 5 servings

1 large butternut squash, halved, peeled, seeded, and cubed

2 red onions, cut into eighths

1 bunch broccolini, or broccoli, 1 inch (2.5 cm) of the base trimmed

4 to 5 bone-in pork chops (1½ to 2 pounds, or 680 to 900 g, total)

3 tablespoons (45 ml) avocado oil

2 tablespoons (28 ml) balsamic vinegar

2 garlic cloves, chopped

1 teaspoon sea salt

4 or 5 thyme sprigs

1. Preheat the oven to 400°F (200°C, or gas mark 6) and line a large baking pan with parchment paper.

2. Place the vegetables and pork chops in the prepared pan. Drizzle with the avocado oil and vinegar. Sprinkle with the garlic and salt and place the thyme on top. Bake for 25 minutes, or until the pork chops reach an internal temperature of 145°F to 150°F (63°C to 66°C) on a meat thermometer. Remove the pork chops from the pan and crisp the vegetables further, if desired, for about 5 minutes.

3. Divide the pork chops and vegetables among four or five plates and serve.

NOTES

To make this meal-prep ready, refrigerate leftovers in individual glass containers for three days. Save some prep time by buying precut butternut squash.

BISCUITS AND SAUSAGE GRAVY

Now *this* is some serious comfort food! In addition to enjoying the biscuits with the homemade sausage gravy, make them whenever you need a bread alternative.

PREP TIME 15 minutes **COOK TIME** 30 minutes **YIELD** Makes 6 servings

FOR THE BISCUITS

⅓ cup (68 g) palm shortening, plus more for preparing the baking sheet.

1 cup (240 ml) coconut milk

1 tablespoon (15 ml) apple cider vinegar

1 cup (140 g) cassava flour

½ cup (56 g) coconut flour

½ teaspoon sea salt

½ teaspoon baking soda

2 teaspoons honey

FOR THE SAUSAGE GRAVY

1 pound (455 g) ground pork

2 teaspoons dried parsley

1 teaspoon dried sage

1 teaspoon garlic powder

½ teaspoon sea salt

Coconut oil, as needed

3 tablespoons (26.5 g) cassava flour

2 cups (475 ml) coconut milk

1. To make the biscuits: Preheat the oven to 400°F (200°C, or gas mark 6).
Line a baking sheet with parchment paper and lightly coat it with palm shortening.

2. In a small bowl, combine the coconut milk and vinegar and set aside.

3. In a large bowl, stir together the cassava and coconut flours, salt, and baking soda until well combined.

4. Cut the palm shortening into the dry ingredients until the mixture forms small pieces.

5. Pour in the honey and coconut milk mixture and stir until all ingredients are well incorporated and a dough forms. Form the dough into six biscuits and place them on the prepared baking sheet, evenly spaced. Bake for 25 to 30 minutes or until cooked through.

6. To make the sausage gravy: While the biscuits cook, in a large deep skillet over medium heat, combine the ground pork, parsley, sage, garlic, and salt and stir to combine. Cook for 7 to 10 minutes, or until browned, breaking up the meat with the back of a spoon. Using a slotted spoon, remove the meat, leaving the fat in the skillet. If you have less than 2 tablespoons (28 ml), add more fat to the pan, preferably coconut oil.

7. Lower the heat, add the cassava flour to the fat, and whisk until thickened.

8. Pour in the coconut milk and whisk until the liquid thickens.

9. Add the cooked pork back to the skillet and stir to combine and heat through. Serve over the biscuits.

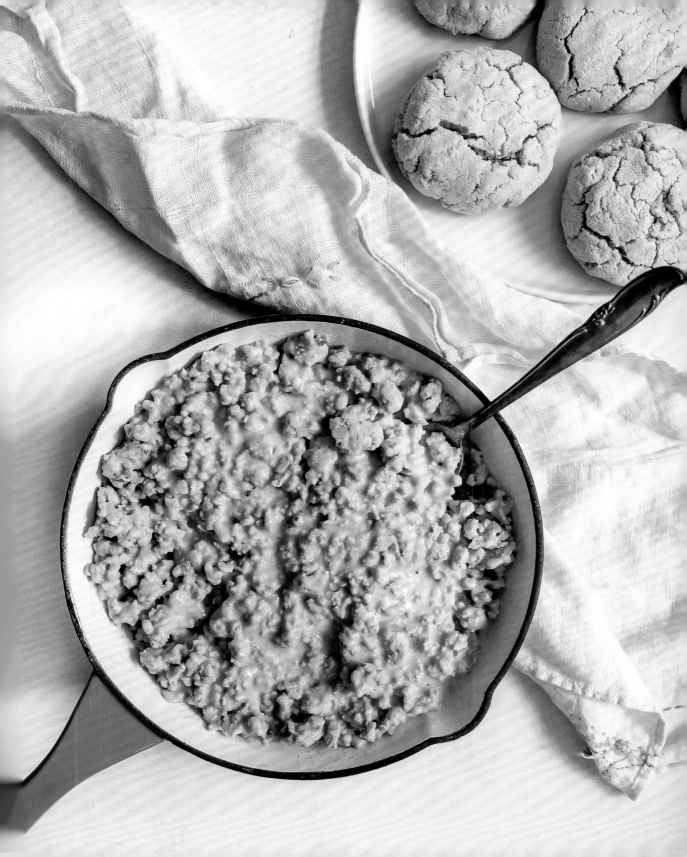

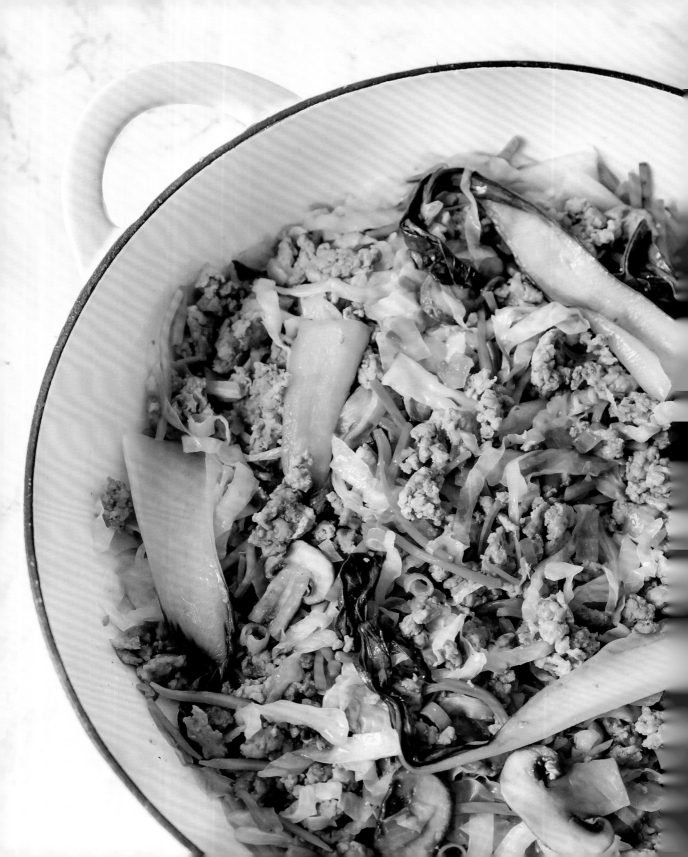

ONE-PAN EGG ROLL

Craving the classic flavors of an egg roll but without the wrapper? This one-pan version is an incredibly simple meal that's made with a variety of vegetables and tastes just like a traditional egg roll.

PREP TIME 15 minutes   **COOK TIME** 25 minutes   **YIELD** Makes 4 servings

1 pound (455 g) ground pork

1 teaspoon sea salt, divided

2 tablespoons (28 g) coconut oil

1 white onion, diced

1 garlic clove, minced

2 teaspoons grated peeled fresh ginger

1 cup (110 g) shredded carrot

2 heads baby bok choy, base trimmed

1 medium head green cabbage, shredded

1 cup (70 g) mushrooms, sliced

2 tablespoons apple cider vinegar

3 tablespoons (45 ml) coconut aminos

2 tablespoons (12 g) chopped scallion

1. In a large skillet over medium heat, combine the ground pork and ¾ teaspoon of salt. Cook for 7 to 8 minutes or until browned, breaking up the meat with the back of a spoon. Remove from the skillet and set aside. Discard the fat and return the skillet to medium heat.

2. Add the coconut oil to the skillet to melt.

3. Add the onion, garlic, and ginger and sauté for 5 to 6 minutes or until the onion is translucent.

4. Add the carrot and sauté for 2 to 3 minutes.

5. Add the bok choy, cabbage, and mushroom and stir to combine.

6. Stir in the vinegar, coconut aminos, and remaining ¼ teaspoon of salt. Cook, stirring, for 4 to 5 minutes to cook down the cabbage.

7. Stir in the pork and cook for 1 minute more or until warmed.

8. Remove from heat and serve warm topped with the scallion.

NOTES

To make this meal-prep ready, refrigerate in individual glass containers for three to four days.

BEEF LIVER & ONIONS

Don't knock it until you try it! Beef liver is a nutritious powerhouse packed with B vitamins and minerals. It pairs well with onion in the classic combination. For the best flavor and the most nutrients, use grass-fed liver.

PREP TIME 1 hour   **COOK TIME** 25 minutes   **YIELD** Makes 3 to 4 servings

1 pound (455 g) grass-fed beef liver

1 cup (240 ml) coconut milk

Juice of 1 lemon

3 bacon slices, chopped

2 apples (Gala or Honeycrisp), peeled and chopped

1 yellow onion, halved and thinly sliced

2 garlic cloves, chopped

3 to 4 tablespoons (45 to 60 ml) avocado oil, divided

½ teaspoon sea salt

1 tablespoon (2 g) fresh rosemary leaves, chopped

1. In a large bowl, submerge the beef liver in the coconut milk and add the lemon juice. This helps remove any bitterness. Refrigerate for 1 hour and drain.

2. In a large deep pan over medium heat, cook the bacon until crispy. Remove the bacon, leaving 2 tablespoons (28 ml) of bacon fat in the pan. Return the pan to medium heat.

3. Add the apples to the bacon fat and cook for about 5 minutes or until soft. Set aside with the bacon.

4. Add the onion and garlic to the pan and cook for 5 to 6 minutes, or until the onion is translucent. Add 1 to 2 tablespoons (15 to 28 ml) of avocado oil, if needed, to prevent burning. Remove the onion and garlic from the pan and set aside, and remove the pan from the heat.

5. Remove the liver from the lemon milk and pat dry. Cut it into cubes and season all sides with salt.

6. Add the remaining 1 to 2 tablespoons (15 to 28 ml) of avocado oil to the pan and place it over medium heat. Add the liver and cook for about 5 minutes or until the internal temperature reaches 160°F (71°C) on a meat thermometer.

7. Add the bacon, apples, and onions to the liver and sprinkle with the rosemary. Cook for about 1 minute more to reheat before serving.

LAMB GYRO SKILLET

Do you love Mediterranean flavors? Same here. Make a fast and flavorful dinner with this lamb gyro skillet! It's made with simple ingredients and seasoned with classic Greek herbs.

PREP TIME 15 minutes   **COOK TIME** 25 minutes   **YIELD** Makes 3 to 4 servings

FOR THE TZATZIKI (OPTIONAL)

½ cup (70 g) Coconut Yogurt (page 37), or store-bought

Juice of ½ lemon

½ cucumber, chopped

1 teaspoon fresh dill

1 teaspoon chopped fresh parsley

¼ teaspoon sea salt, plus more as needed

FOR THE LAMB SKILLET

1 pound (455 g) ground lamb

1 teaspoon sea salt, divided

2 garlic cloves, minced

2 cups (200 g) Basic Cauliflower Rice (page 28)

1 zucchini, halved and cut into half-moons

1 medium red onion, chopped

1 tablespoon (4 g) chopped fresh parsley

1 teaspoon fresh dill

Juice of ½ lemon

8 to 12 olives

1. To make the tzatziki (if using): In a small bowl, whisk all the ingredients. Taste, adjust the seasoning, and set aside.

2. To make the lamb skillet: In a large skillet over medium heat, combine the ground lamb and ½ teaspoon of salt. Cook for about 7 minutes until browned and cooked through, breaking up the meat with the back of a spoon. Using a slotted spoon, remove the meat, leaving 2 tablespoons (28 ml) of fat in the skillet. Return the skillet to medium heat.

3. Add the garlic to the skillet and cook for 2 to 3 minutes, or until fragrant.

4. Add the cauliflower rice, zucchini, and red onion and cook for 7 to 8 minutes, or until tender.

5. Return the lamb to the skillet and top with the parsley, dill, remaining ½ teaspoon of salt, and the lemon juice. Stir well. Cook for 2 to 3 minutes to reheat and let the flavors combine. Serve topped with the olives and tzatziki (if using).

NOTES

To make this meal-prep ready, refrigerate in individual glass containers, with the tzatziki in a separate container, for three to four days.

ZUCCHINI CHICKEN ENCHILADAS

Can you really make enchiladas without nightshade spices, cheese, or a corn or flour tortilla? Yes! These zucchini enchiladas are a veggie-packed Sunday dinner that's so much fun to eat. If your household is anything like ours, one pan of these enchiladas won't make it past the 24-hour mark. However, they also make a great meal-prep option.

PREP TIME 15 minutes   **COOK TIME** 45 minutes   **YIELD** 10 to 12 enchiladas

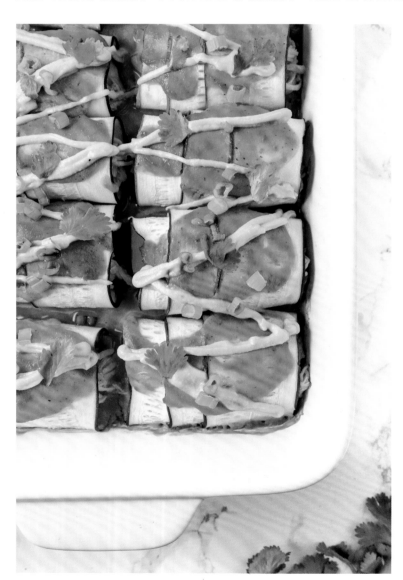

FOR THE ENCHILADA SAUCE

2 tablespoons (28 ml) avocado oil

1 medium white onion, finely diced

1 cup (250 g) Nightshade-free "Tomato" Sauce (page 31)

½ cup (120 ml) Chicken Bone Broth (page 24)

½ cup (120 ml) water

2 to 3 teaspoons (4 to 7 g) horseradish powder

2 teaspoons garlic powder

¾ teaspoon sea salt

FOR THE AVOCADO SOUR CREAM

2 avocados

¼ cup (60 ml) avocado oil

Juice of 1 lime

½ teaspoon sea salt

FOR THE ENCHILADAS

1 pound (455 g) shredded cooked chicken breast

4 to 5 large zucchini, ends trimmed

2 tablespoons (2 g) chopped fresh cilantro

2 tablespoons (12 g) sliced scallion

1. To make the enchilada sauce: In a medium saucepan over medium heat, heat the avocado oil.

2. Add the onion and sauté for 5 to 6 minutes or until lightly translucent.

3. Stir in the remaining ingredients and bring to a simmer. Cook for 10 to 15 minutes, stirring occasionally, or until the sauce thickens. If you prefer a smoother sauce, use an immersion blender to blend the sauce until smooth. Set aside.

4. Preheat the oven to 350°F (180°C, or gas mark 4).

5. To make the enchiladas: Layer one-third of the enchilada sauce on the bottom of a 9 x 13-inch (23 x 33 cm) baking dish and mix another one-third with the chicken. Set aside.

6. Using a vegetable peeler or mandoline set to ⅛ inch (3 mm), slice long, thin, vertical slices of zucchini. Set aside for 5 minutes and then pat dry with a paper towel or clean dishtowel.

7. While the zucchini rests, make the avocado cream: In a high-speed blender, combine all the ingredients for the cream and blend until smooth.

8. To assemble the enchiladas: On your work surface, line up three "sheets" of zucchini so they're barely overlapping. Place about ¼ cup (35 g) of the shredded chicken mixture near one end of the "sheet" and roll the zucchini up and around until you have a wrapped enchilada. Place the enchilada in the baking dish. Repeat until you have filled the baking dish with about 10 to 12 enchiladas. Top with the remainder of the enchilada sauce. Bake for 15 to 20 minutes. Set aside to cool.

9. Top the enchiladas with the avocado sour cream, cilantro, and scallion before serving.

NOTES

To make this meal-prep ready, leave the Avocado Sour Cream off and when ready, serve with fresh avocado to avoid browning.

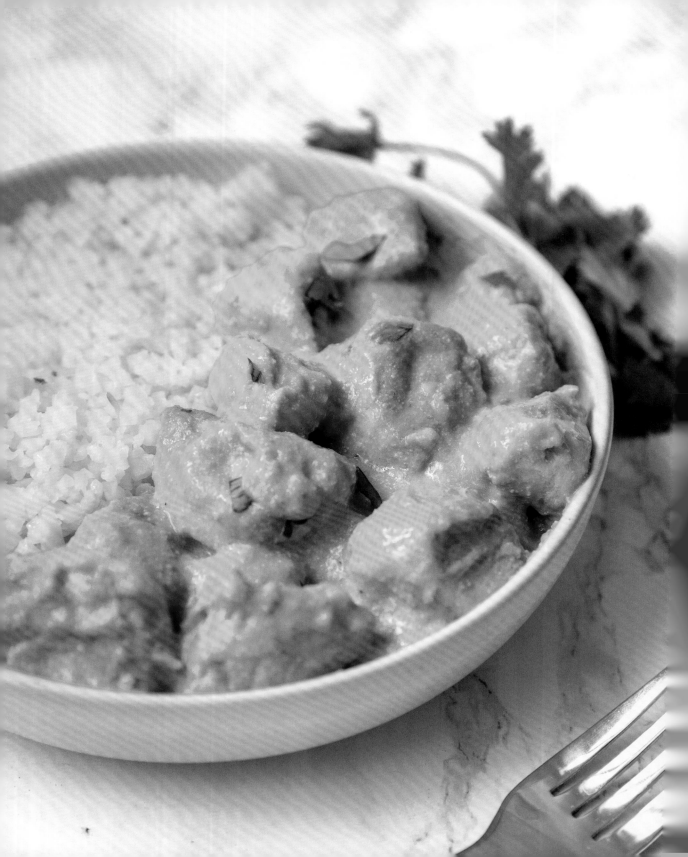

CHICKEN TIKKA MASALA

This dish is creamy, flavorful, and absolutely delicious! Though it's a bit more prep work than some of the other recipes in this book, it's worth it. Save a few steps by buying coconut yogurt at the store (see Notes) and using Night-shade-Free "Tomato" Sauce (page 31) that was prepped ahead of time and stored in the freezer.

PREP TIME 4 hours   **COOK TIME** 40 minutes   **YIELD** Makes 4 servings

FOR THE CHICKEN AND MARINADE

1 cup (170 g) Coconut Yogurt (page 37), or store-bought

Juice of ½ lemon

1 teaspoon ground turmeric

½ teaspoon horseradish powder

½ teaspoon sea salt

1½ pounds (680 g) boneless chicken breast, cubed

FOR THE SAUCE

1 tablespoon (14 g) coconut oil

1 medium onion, diced

2 teaspoons ground turmeric

1 teaspoon ground ginger

½ teaspoon sea salt

2 cups (500 g) Nightshade-Free "Tomato" Sauce (page 31)

1 cup (240 g) coconut cream

FOR SERVING

1 tablespoon (1 g) chopped fresh cilantro

2 to 3 (200 to 300 g) cups Basic Cauliflower Rice (page 28)

1. To make the chicken and marinade: In a medium bowl, whisk the coconut yogurt, lemon juice, turmeric, horseradish powder, and salt until combined. Add the chicken, turn to coat with the marinade, cover, and refrigerate for 3 to 4 hours or overnight.

2. Place a deep skillet over medium heat. Remove the chicken from the marinade and add it to the skillet. Sauté for 8 to 10 minutes or until the internal temperature reaches 165°F (74°C) on a meat thermometer. Remove the chicken and set aside.

3. To make the sauce: Return the skillet to medium heat and add the coconut oil to melt.

4. Add the onion and sauté for 5 to 6 minutes. Stir in the turmeric, ginger, and salt.

5. Stir in the "tomato" sauce and bring to a low simmer. Reduce the heat to medium-low and cook for 15 to 20 minutes, or until the sauce thickens into a paste. Stir in the coconut cream, mixing well.

6. Add the chicken to the sauce and cook for a few minutes to reheat the chicken and combine the flavors.

7. To serve: Serve the chicken over the cauliflower rice, garnished with cilantro.

NOTES

If you use store-bought coconut yogurt, be sure there are no added sugars or thickeners such as xanthan or guar gum.

ONE-PAN CHICKEN PICCATA WITH ASPARAGUS

Chicken piccata is a delicious Italian dish that's typically made with floured chicken and a sauce containing white wine, lemon, and capers. Though the alcohol is generally cooked out, this recipe still omits the wine.

PREP TIME 10 minutes   **COOK TIME** 20 minutes   **YIELD** Makes 5 to 6 servings

1 pound (455 g) chicken cutlets (see Notes)

1 teaspoon sea salt, plus more for seasoning

¼ cup (36 g) arrowroot starch

3 tablespoons (45 ml) avocado oil

2 garlic cloves, minced

1 bunch asparagus, trimmed

1 cup (235 ml) Chicken Bone Broth (page 24)

Juice of 1 large lemon

2 tablespoons (18 g) capers

½ lemon, sliced

1 tablespoon (4 g) chopped fresh parsley

1. Pat the chicken cutlets dry and season both sides with salt.

2. Place the arrowroot starch in a shallow bowl and dredge the chicken in it on both sides.

3. In a large deep pan over medium heat, heat the avocado oil.

4. Add the chicken and cook for 4 to 5 minutes on each side or until the chicken is lightly browned and the internal temperature reaches 165°F (74°C) on a meat thermometer. Remove the chicken.

5. Reduce the heat under the pan slightly and add the garlic. Cook for 2 to 3 minutes or until fragrant.

6. Add the asparagus to the pan and season lightly with salt. Pour in the bone broth and bring to a low simmer. Cover the pan and simmer for 5 minutes or until the asparagus is tender.

7. Return the chicken to the pan and add the lemon juice and capers. Cook for 1 minute to reheat the chicken. Serve topped with lemon slices and parsley.

NOTES

You can buy chicken cutlets prepared at the butcher counter, or you can simply slice a chicken breast in half, lengthwise.

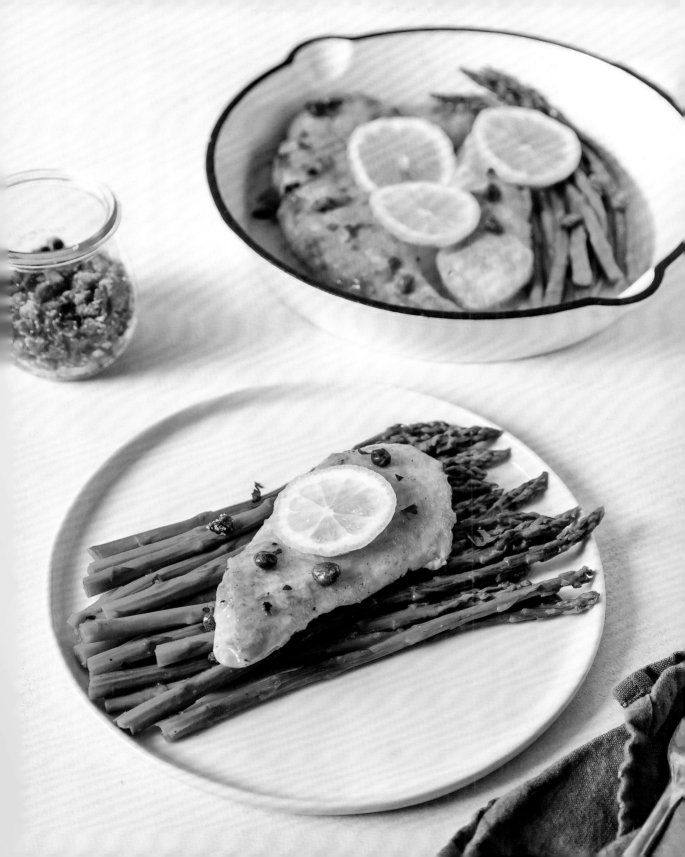

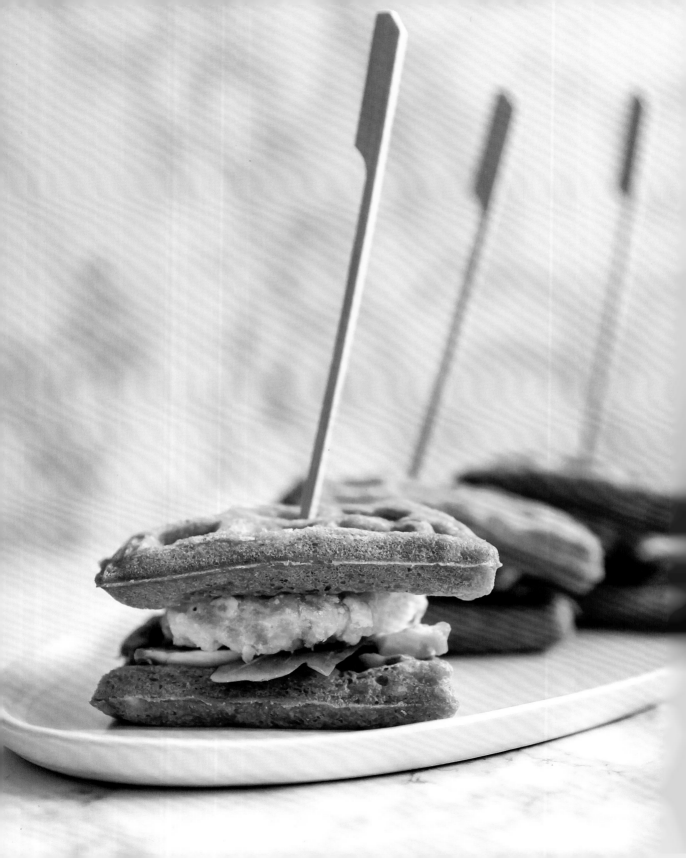

CHICKEN & WAFFLE SANDWICHES

Oh, yes, we're going there! These sandwiches are decadent, comforting, and a seriously yummy special-occasion food. They're hearty enough to enjoy as a main dish, but can be served at brunch or as a filling appetizer.

PREP TIME 1 hour   **COOK TIME** 35 minutes   **YIELD** Makes 3 to 4 servings

1 pound (455 g) boneless chicken breast

1 cup (240 ml) coconut milk

2 tablespoons (30 ml) apple cider vinegar

2 tablespoons (45 ml) avocado oil

3 tablespoons (24 g) arrowroot starch

2 tablespoons (16 g) coconut flour

½ teaspoon dried parsley

2 teaspoons garlic powder

1 teaspoon onion powder

1 teaspoon sea salt

3 or 4 waffles, quartered (see Blueberry Waffles, page 34)

Arugula, for serving

Sliced avocado, for serving

Honey, for serving (optional)

1. Slice the chicken into 6 to 8 pieces (1 for each sandwich), small enough to fit between the quartered waffles, and thin.

2. In a medium bowl, whisk the coconut milk and vinegar and allow to sit for 5 minutes. Add the chicken and mix well to coat all the pieces. Refrigerate for 20 to 25 minutes. Remove and drain the excess liquid.

3. Preheat the oven to 400°F (200°C, or gas mark 6). Line a large baking sheet with parchment paper and set aside.

4. In another medium bowl, stir the dry ingredients together.

5. Working one at a time, dip each piece of chicken into the dry ingredients, thoroughly coating it. Place the coated chicken on the prepared baking sheet. Drizzle with the avocado oil. Bake for 30 to 35 minutes, flipping halfway through the cooking time for even cooking, or until the internal temperature reaches 165°F (74°C) on a meat thermometer.

6. Assemble the sandwiches: On one quarter-waffle piece, place a layer of arugula, avocado, and chicken and top with another waffle piece. Use a small skewer to hold the sandwich together. Repeat to assemble the remaining sandwiches and serve with honey (if desired).

CILANTRO AVOCADO CHICKEN POPPERS

If you've ever read my blog, you may have seen that I have several recipes for chicken poppers! They're easy to make, cost effective, and kid friendly. All my chicken popper recipes feature ground chicken, some sort of starchy vegetable, and other herbs and vegetables for flavor. This version has all those elements, plus whole chunks of avocado to add more healthy fat and flavor!

PREP TIME 15 minutes   **COOK TIME** 25 minutes   **YIELD** Makes 3 to 4 servings

2 cups (266 g) chopped peeled sweet potato

1 pound (455 g) ground chicken (see Notes for substitutions)

2 tablespoons (23 ml) avocado oil

2 tablespoons (14 g) coconut flour

1 tablespoon (1 g) chopped fresh cilantro

1 garlic clove, minced

2 teaspoons onion powder

¾ teaspoon sea salt

Juice of 1 lime

1 medium avocado, peeled, pitted, and diced

Guacamole (page 58), for serving

1. Preheat the oven to 400°F (200°C, or gas mark 6) and line a baking sheet with parchment paper. Set aside.

2. In a food processor, process the sweet potato until it's finely riced and transfer to a large bowl.

3. Add the ground chicken, avocado oil, coconut flour, cilantro, garlic, onion powder, salt, and lime juice. Use your hands to mix well and thoroughly combine the ingredients. Set aside.

4. Take a small handful of the chicken mixture and carefully fold in one to three avocado cubes. Slightly flatten the chicken mixture into poppers and place on the prepared baking sheet. Repeat the process with the remaining ingredients. You should have about 25 poppers. Bake for about 25 minutes, flipping halfway through the baking time, or until the internal temperature reaches 165°F (74°C) on a meat thermometer.

5. If you like a crispier texture, broil for 1 to 2 minutes to crisp further.

6. Serve with guacamole for dipping.

NOTES

If you can't find ground chicken, simply add 1 pound (455 g) of chicken breast to a food processor to make your own! You can also use ground turkey.

To make this coconut free, substitute cassava flour for the coconut flour.

To make meal-prep ready, store in a glass container for 1 to 2 days and serve guacamole fresh.

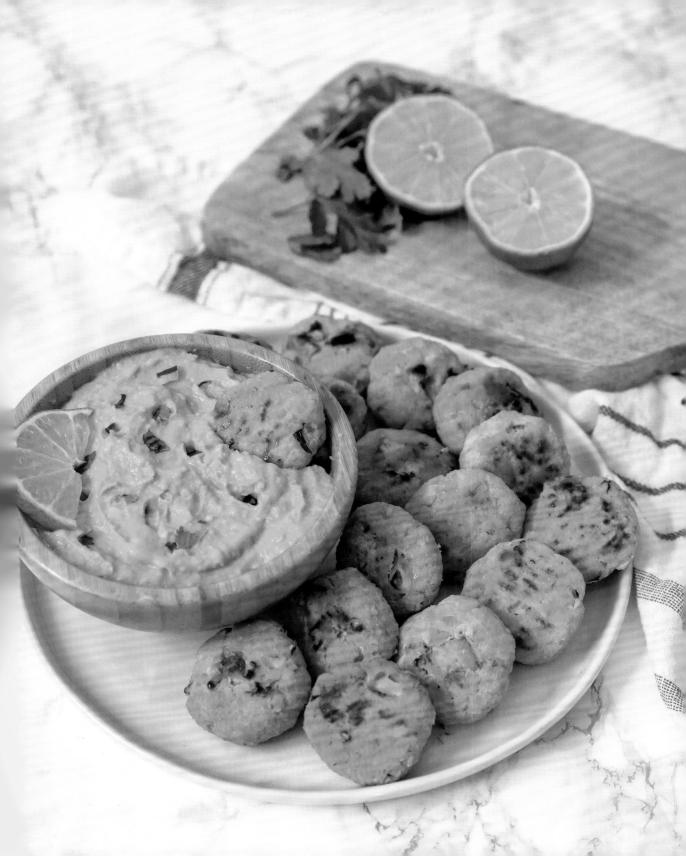

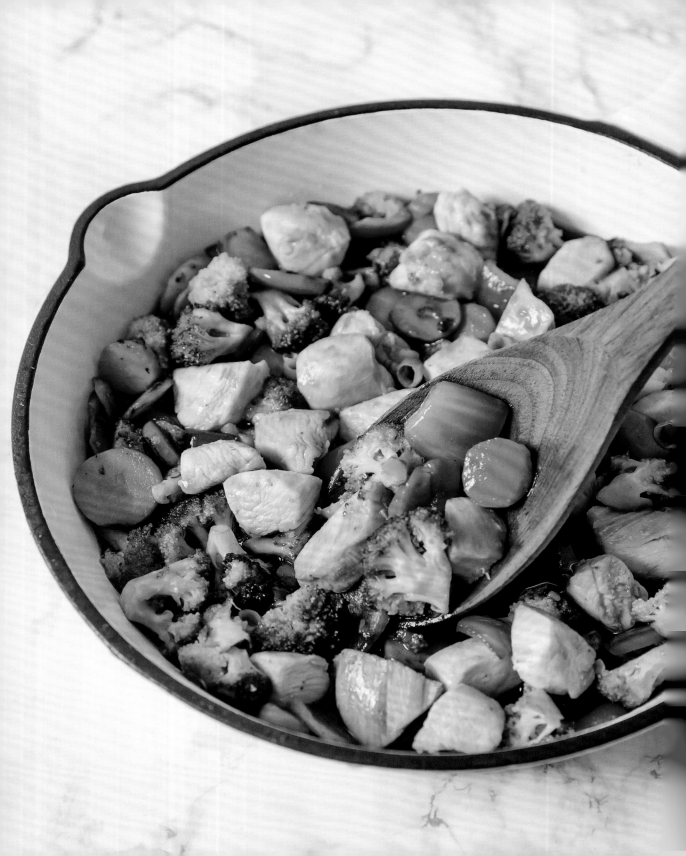

TERIYAKI CHICKEN STIR-FRY

You can never go wrong with a teriyaki chicken stir-fry. It's fast, flavorful, and filling and the ultimate go-to when you're just not sure what to make. My husband and I eat this recipe at least once a week, and it never fails to satisfy.

PREP TIME 15 minutes   **COOK TIME** 25 minutes   **YIELD** Makes 3 to 4 servings

FOR THE SAUCE

¼ cup (60 ml) coconut aminos, plus more as needed

2 tablespoons (28 ml) fresh orange juice

2 teaspoons honey

1 teaspoon grated peeled fresh ginger

1 teaspoon onion powder

½ teaspoon sea salt

1 teaspoon arrowroot starch

FOR THE TERIYAKI CHICKEN

2 to 3 tablespoons (28 to 42 g) coconut oil, or (28 to 45 ml) avocado oil

½ medium red onion, chopped

2 cups (142 g) broccoli florets

1 cup (130 g) chopped carrot

½ teaspoon sea salt, divided

1 pound (455 g) boneless chicken breast, cubed

2 to 3 scallions, sliced

Basic Cauliflower Rice (page 28), for serving (optional)

1. To make the sauce: In a small saucepan over low heat, whisk the coconut aminos, orange juice, honey, ginger, onion powder, and salt. Cook for 3 to 4 minutes.

2. Whisk in the arrowroot starch. Cook for 2 minutes more to thicken. Add more coconut aminos for a thinner consistency, if desired. Set aside.

3. To make the teriyaki chicken: In a large deep skillet over medium heat, melt the coconut oil.

4. Add the red onion, broccoli, carrot, and ¼ teaspoon of salt. Cook for about 7 minutes or until the vegetables are tender. Using a slotted spoon, remove the vegetables, leaving the fat in the skillet. Return the skillet to medium heat.

5. Add the chicken and lightly season with the remaining ¼ teaspoon of salt. Cook for 5 to 7 minutes or until the internal temperature reaches 165°F (74°C) on a meat thermometer.

6. Add the vegetables and sauce to the pan and stir to combine. Cook for about 1 minute to heat through and add the scallion. Serve with the cauliflower rice (if using).

NOTES

To make this meal-prep ready, refrigerate in individual glass containers for three to four days to enjoy throughout the week.

EASY HAWAIIAN CHICKEN DINNER

This meal is easy to make and can be eaten by itself or with a simple side, such as Basic Cauliflower Rice (page 28) or a small salad. It's also a great meal prep option to make on a Sunday, refrigerate in individual glass containers, and enjoy throughout the week.

PREP TIME 5 minutes   **COOK TIME** 35 minutes   **YIELD** Makes 4 servings

FOR THE SAUCE

5 tablespoons (75 ml) pineapple juice

3 tablespoons (45 ml) coconut aminos, plus more as needed

¾ teaspoon sea salt

1½ teaspoons arrowroot starch

FOR THE HAWAIIAN CHICKEN

1½ pounds (680 g) boneless chicken breast, cubed

2 cups (330 g) cubed pineapple

2 cups (142 g) chopped broccoli

1 large red onion, roughly chopped

2 tablespoons (28 g) coconut oil, melted

1 tablespoon (1 g) chopped fresh cilantro

2 to 3 scallions, sliced

1. To make the sauce: In a small saucepan over low heat, whisk the pineapple juice, coconut aminos, and salt. Cook for 3 to 4 minutes.

2. Whisk in the arrowroot starch. Cook for 2 minutes more to thicken. Add more coconut aminos for a thinner consistency, if desired. Set aside.

3. To make the Hawaiian chicken: Preheat the oven to 375°F (190°C, or gas mark 5) and line a large baking sheet with parchment paper. Set aside.

4. In a large bowl, combine the sauce, chicken, pineapple, broccoli, red onion, and melted coconut oil, stirring until the chicken is completely coated. Transfer the mixture to the prepared baking sheet in an even layer. Bake for 30 minutes or until the chicken reaches an internal temperature of 165°F (74°C) on a meat thermometer.

5. Top with the cilantro and scallion. Serve immediately.

NOTES

To make this meal-prep ready, cool before refrigerating in individual glass containers to eat throughout the week.

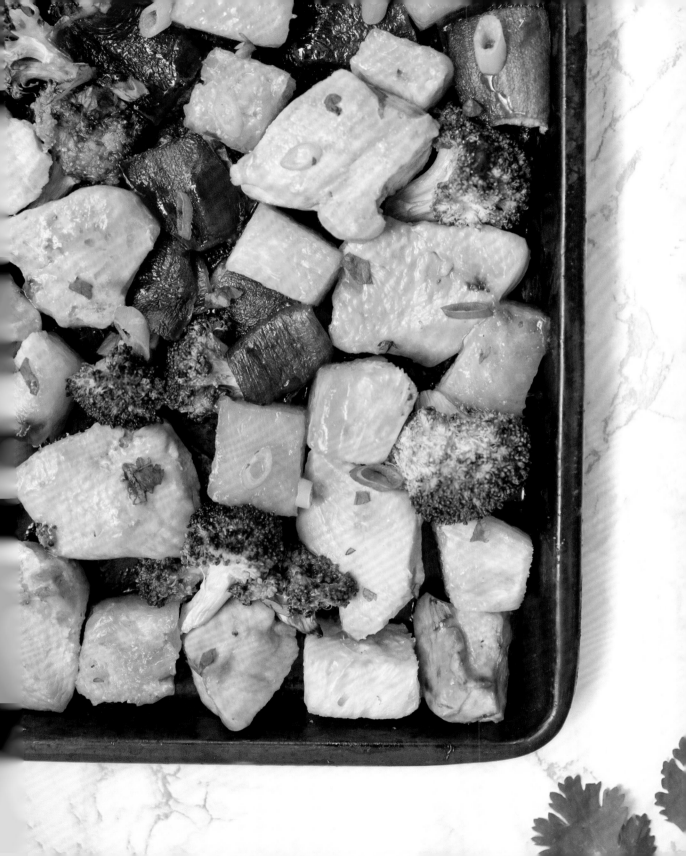

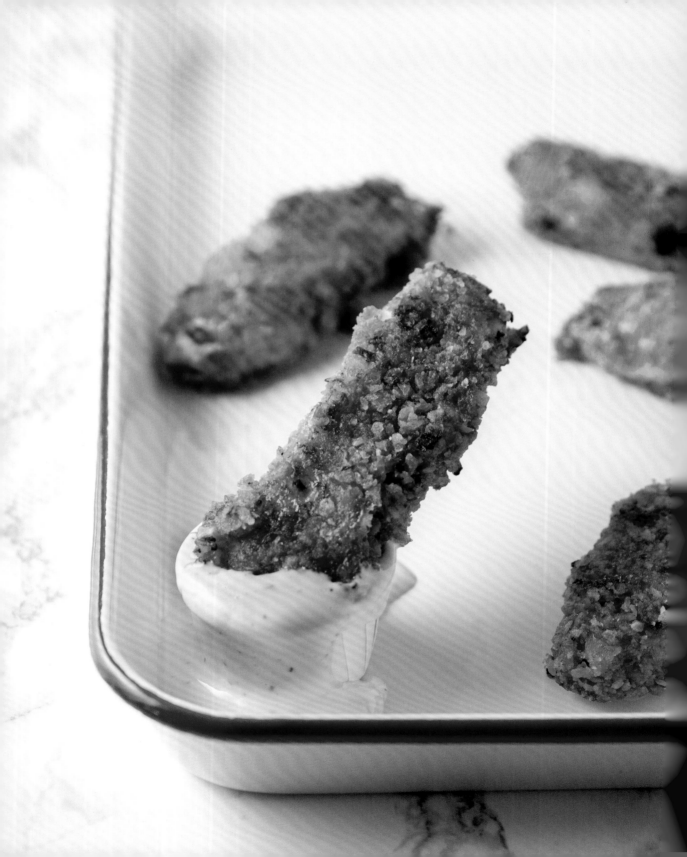

HONEY "BUTTERMILK" CHICKEN STRIPS WITH RANCH DIP

I grew up eating chicken nuggets and chicken strips *several* times a week and consider myself a bit of an enthusiast. This recipe makes them AIP compliant without losing any of the flavor of the traditional version.

PREP TIME 1 hour, 10 minutes   **COOK TIME** 30 minutes   **YIELD** Makes 2 to 3 servings

FOR THE RANCH DIP

⅓ cup (80 g) coconut cream (see Notes)

3 tablespoons (45 ml) coconut milk (see Notes)

2 teaspoons apple cider vinegar

2 teaspoons chopped fresh parsley

1 teaspoon chopped fresh chives

½ teaspoon dried dill

½ teaspoon garlic powder

½ teaspoon onion powder

½ teaspoon sea salt

FOR THE CHICKEN STRIPS

1 cup (235 ml) coconut milk

¼ cup (80 g) honey

2 tablespoons (28 ml) apple cider vinegar

1 pound (455 g) boneless chicken breast, cut into strips

3 cups (114 g) Plantain Chips (page 59)

1 tablespoon (3 g) chopped fresh chives

¼ teaspoon sea salt

⅓ cup (75 g) coconut oil, melted

1. To make the ranch dip: In a medium bowl, whisk the coconut cream, coconut milk, and vinegar until creamy and fully combined. Whisk in the seasonings. Refrigerate until needed.

2. To make the chicken strips: In another medium bowl, stir together the coconut milk, honey, and vinegar. Allow to sit for 5 minutes. Add the chicken, stirring well to coat. Cover and refrigerate for 45 to 60 minutes. Remove and drain the excess milk.

3. Preheat the oven to 400°F (200°C, or gas mark 6) and line a large baking sheet with parchment paper.

4. In a food processor, grind the plantain chips until fine. Transfer to a medium bowl and stir in the chives and salt.

5. Place the coconut oil in another bowl and place it next to the chip mixture.

6. Using tongs, dip each chicken strip into the coconut oil and then the plantain mixture. Place the coated strips on the prepared baking sheet. Bake for 20 to 25 minutes, carefully flipping them halfway through the baking time. Transfer to a plate and let cool for about 10 minutes. Serve with the ranch dip.

NOTES

For the ranch dip, place a can of coconut milk in the refrigerator overnight and use the cream that hardens on the top and the water that settles on the bottom.

The coating on the chicken strips is delicate, so be careful when flipping and transferring. The chicken strips need time to cool so the coating sets before eating.

BACON RANCH TURKEY BURGERS

These turkey burgers are flavored with a homemade ranch seasoning and topped with a creamy avocado ranch dressing and crispy bacon! They're a unique addition to any barbecue, but easy enough to make on a weeknight.

PREP TIME 10 minutes **COOK TIME** 20 minutes **YIELD** Makes 4 burgers

FOR THE AVOCADO RANCH

1 large avocado, pitted and peeled

3 to 4 tablespoons (45 to 60 ml) coconut milk (see Notes)

1 tablespoon (15 ml) avocado oil

2 teaspoons apple cider vinegar

2 teaspoons chopped fresh parsley

1 teaspoon chopped fresh chives

½ teaspoon dried dill

½ teaspoon onion powder

½ teaspoon garlic powder

½ teaspoon sea salt

FOR THE TURKEY BURGERS

1 pound (455 g) ground turkey

2 tablespoons (8 g) chopped fresh parsley

2 teaspoons chopped fresh chives

2 teaspoons onion powder

2 teaspoons garlic powder

1 teaspoon fresh dill

¾ teaspoon sea salt

1 tablespoon (7 g) coconut flour

1 tablespoon (14 g) coconut oil, plus more for preparing the grill pan

4 to 5 bacon slices, cooked

½ medium red onion, sliced

1 head green leaf lettuce or butter lettuce, leaves separated

1. To make the avocado ranch: Scoop the avocado flesh into a high-speed blender, add the remaining ingredients, and blend until smooth. Set aside.

2. To make the turkey burgers: In a large bowl, mix together the ground turkey, parsley, chives, onion powder, garlic powder, dill, salt, coconut flour, and coconut oil until fully combined. Form the mixture into four turkey burgers and set aside.

3. Lightly coat a grill pan or cast iron pan with coconut oil and place it over high heat until hot.

4. Two at a time, add the burgers to the pan. Grill for about 5 minutes on each side or until the internal temperature reaches 165°F (74°C) on a meat thermometer. Remove from the heat and let cool slightly. Repeat with the remaining burgers.

5. Assemble the turkey burgers by topping with the avocado ranch, bacon, and red onions. Serve alone or wrapped in a lettuce leaf.

NOTES

The amount of coconut milk used will vary depending on the size of your avocado, and how creamy you'd like the ranch to be. Add 1 tablespoon (15 ml) more or less, as needed.

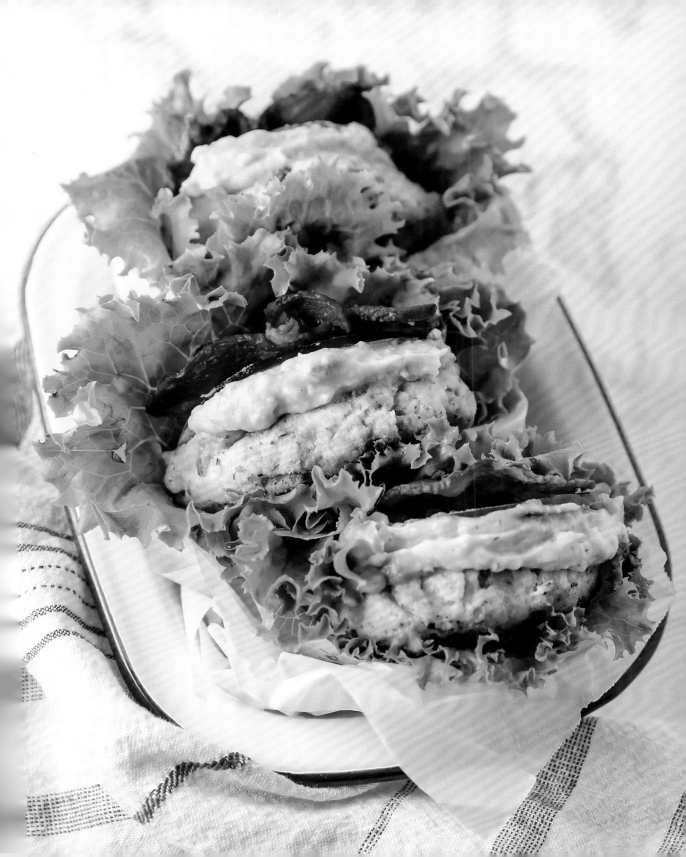

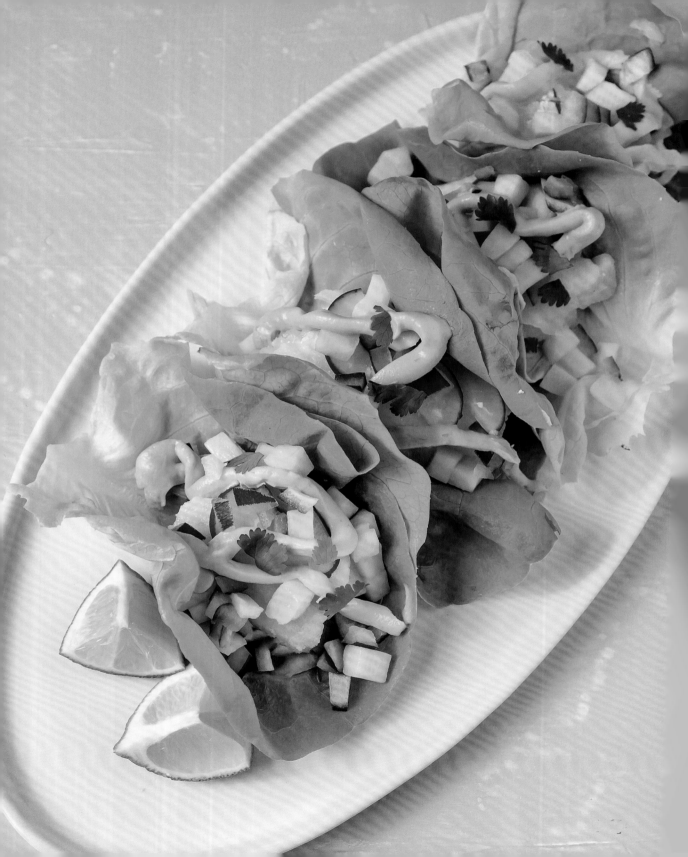

BAJA FISH TACOS

These fish tacos help you add more greens to your day and save time on making tortillas by using butter lettuce as the taco shell.

PREP TIME 15 minutes   **COOK TIME** 5 minutes   **YIELD** Makes 2 servings

¼ cup (60 ml) avocado oil

3 tablespoons (27 g) arrowroot starch

2 (5 to 6 ounce [140 to 170 g] cod fillets

½ teaspoon sea salt

4 butter lettuce leaves

¼ cup (44 g) diced mango

½ cup (80 g) diced red onion

2 radishes, halved and sliced

2 to 3 tablespoons (30 to 45 g) Avocado Sour Cream (page 124), or 1 avocado, pitted, peeled, and diced

1 tablespoon (1 g) chopped fresh cilantro

1 lime, quartered

1. In a large deep pan over medium-high heat, heat the avocado oil.

2. Place the arrowroot starch in a shallow bowl. Season the cod fillets on both sides with salt and dredge them in the starch. Carefully place the fillets in the pan. Cook for 2 to 3 minutes on each side, carefully flipping in between. Set aside and cut in half.

3. Place the butter lettuce leaves on a work surface. Evenly dividing the ingredients, layer on the cod, mango, red onion, and radish slices. Top with the avocado sour cream (or fresh avocado) and cilantro. Serve immediately with a lime wedge for squeezing.

SHRIMP ALFREDO

There's nothing quite like a creamy Alfredo sauce! This recipe offers a veggie-packed alternative to the traditional heavy Alfredo, but still retains its creaminess.

PREP TIME 15 minutes   **COOK TIME** 1 hour   **YIELD** Makes 8 to 9 servings

FOR THE SPAGHETTI SQUASH

1 medium spaghetti squash, halved lengthwise, seeded

FOR THE ALFREDO SAUCE

4 cups (400 g) cauliflower florets

½ cup (120 ml) coconut milk

¼ cup (60 ml) Chicken Bone Broth (page 25)

1 tablespoon (4 g) nutritional yeast

1 tablespoon (15 ml) olive oil

1 garlic clove, peeled

¼ teaspoon sea salt

FOR THE SHRIMP

2 tablespoons (28 ml) olive oil

12 ounces (340 g) medium shrimp, peeled and deveined

½ teaspoon sea salt

1 tablespoon (4 g) chopped fresh parsley

1. To make the spaghetti squash: Preheat the oven to 400°F (200°C, or gas mark 6) and line a baking sheet with parchment paper.

2. Place the squash halves skin-side up on the prepared baking sheet. Bake for 40 to 50 minutes or until the skin is soft.

3. Let cool slightly before using a fork to pull the strands out of the squash. Set the strands aside and discard the skin.

4. To make the alfredo sauce: While the squash cooks, fill a medium pot with about 2 inches (5 cm) of water and add the cauliflower. Place the pot over medium heat and bring to a low simmer. Cover the pot and cook for 8 to 10 minutes, or until the cauliflower is soft. Strain and use a paper towel or cheesecloth to remove any excess moisture. Transfer to a high-speed blender. Add the remaining sauce ingredients and blend until smooth. Set aside.

5. To make the shrimp: In a large deep pan over medium-low heat, heat the olive oil.

6. Season the shrimp with salt and add them to the pan. Cook for about 2 minutes on each side or until pink. Remove from the pan. Return the skillet to the heat.

7. Add the squash and Alfredo sauce and heat for 1 to 2 minutes. Fold the shrimp into the squash, top with the parsley, and serve immediately.

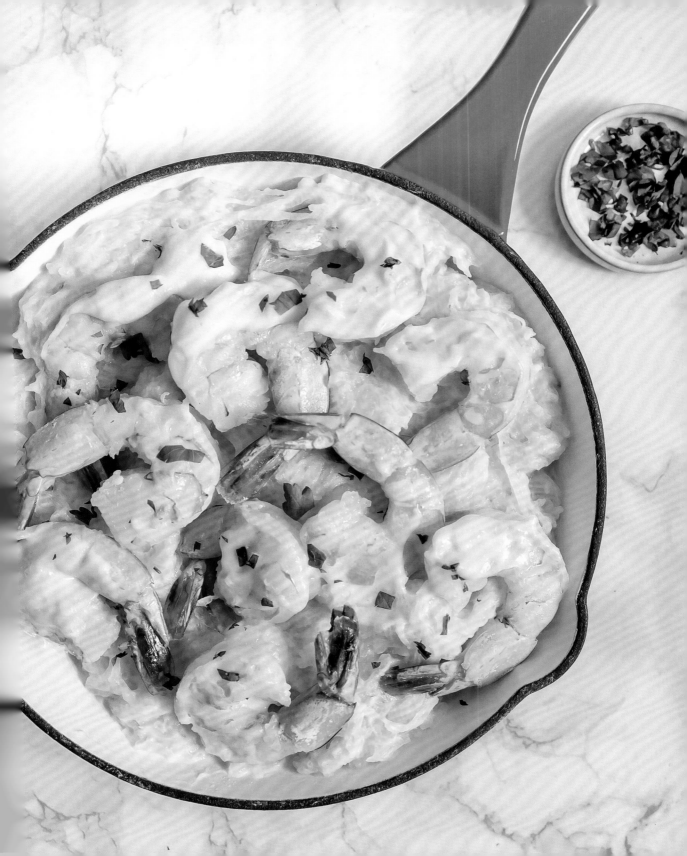

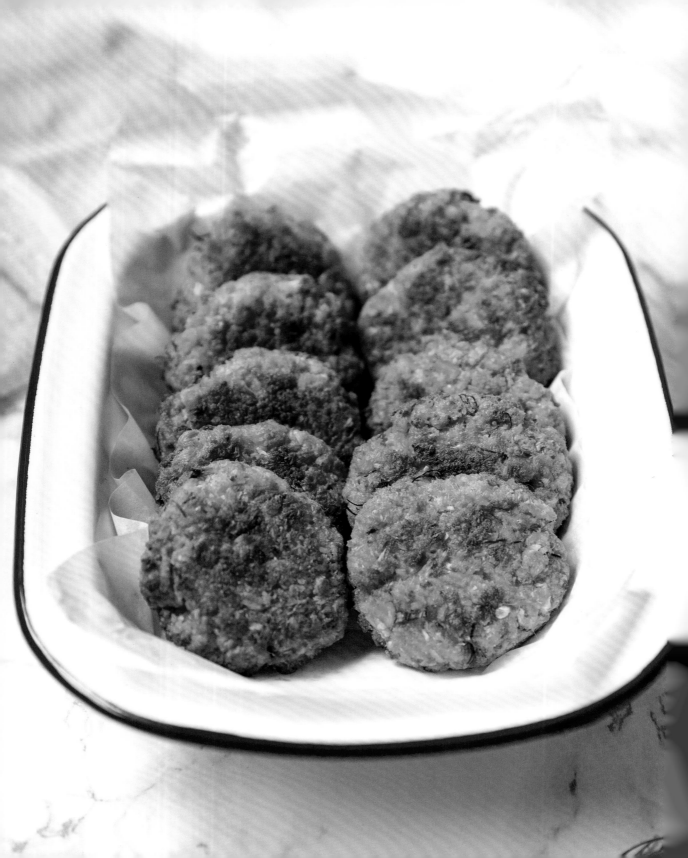

HERBED SALMON CAKES

These salmon cakes are packed with veggies, protein, and healthy fats! They're the perfect way to squeeze in some nutrient-dense ingredients disguised as crispy comfort food.

PREP TIME 20 minutes   **COOK TIME** 45 minutes   **YIELD** Makes 8 to 10 salmon cakes

1 heaping cup (120 g) chopped zucchini

½ cup (65 g) chopped carrot

2 tablespoons (12 g) chopped scallion

1 tablespoon (4 g) chopped fresh parsley

1 tablespoon (7 g) coconut flour

1 tablespoon (9 g) arrowroot starch

1 teaspoon dried dill

½ teaspoon sea salt

1 can (6 ounce [170 g]) can salmon, drained

1 tablespoon (15 ml) fresh lemon juice

2 tablespoons (28 g) coconut oil

1. Preheat the oven to 400°F (200°C, or gas mark 6) and line a baking sheet with parchment paper. Set aside.

2. In a food processor, combine the zucchini and carrot and process until shredded and no large pieces remain. Transfer to a nut milk bag or wrap in cheesecloth or paper towel and squeeze to drain the excess water. Put the vegetables in a large bowl.

3. Stir in the scallion, parsley, coconut flour, arrowroot starch, dill, and salt.

4. Using your hands, squeeze any excess liquid from the drained salmon and add it to the bowl along with the lemon juice and coconut oil. Using your hands, mix the ingredients until fully combined. Form the mixture into seven or eight flattened salmon cakes about 2 inches (5 cm) in diameter and place them on the prepared baking sheet. Bake for 40 to 45 minutes, carefully flipping them halfway through the baking time.

5. Let cool before serving.

NOTES

To make this meal-prep ready, refrigerate in an airtight glass container for one to two days. These salmon cakes also taste great cold!

SHRIMP & GRITS WITH SPINACH

This Southern classic is traditionally made with ingredients that are far from AIP compliant, such as nightshade spices, corn, and butter. This version is made with an AIP-friendly spice blend and nutrient-dense vegetables.

PREP TIME 15 minutes   **COOK TIME** 30 minutes   **YIELD** Makes 2 servings

FOR THE CAULIFLOWER GRITS
2½ cups (250 g) cauliflower, riced

2 tablespoons (28 g) coconut oil

2 tablespoons (30 ml) coconut milk

2 teaspoons garlic powder

½ teaspoon sea salt

FOR THE SPINACH
1 tablespoon (14 g) coconut oil

3 cups (90 g) spinach

¼ teaspoon sea salt

FOR THE SHRIMP
2 teaspoons garlic powder

2 teaspoons onion powder

1 teaspoon sea salt

1 teaspoon dried thyme

1 teaspoon dried oregano

¼ teaspoon ground turmeric

1 pound (455 g) medium shrimp, peeled and deveined

2 to 3 tablespoons (28 to 42 g) coconut oil

Juice of ½ lemon

1 tablespoon (4 g) chopped fresh parsley

1. To make the cauliflower grits: In a medium pot, combine the cauliflower rice and enough water just to cover. Place the pot over medium heat and bring to a low simmer. Cover the pot and steam for about 7 minutes, or until the cauliflower rice is soft. Strain the excess water from the pot. Transfer the cauliflower rice to a food processor.

2. Add the coconut oil, coconut milk, garlic powder, and salt to the processor. Blend until smooth. Divide evenly among two plates or bowls and set aside.

3. To make the spinach: In a skillet over medium heat, melt the coconut oil.

4. Add the spinach and salt. Cook for 3 to 4 minutes or until the spinach is wilted. Divide the spinach over the cauliflower grits.

5. To make the shrimp: In a medium bowl, stir together the garlic powder, onion powder, salt, thyme, oregano, and turmeric.

6. Add the shrimp and toss to coat generously.

7. In a large deep pan over medium heat, melt the coconut oil.

8. Working in two or three batches so as not to crowd the pan, add the coated shrimp and cook for about 2 minutes on each side or until the shrimp turn pink. Place the shrimp over the grits and spinach. Sprinkle with the lemon juice and garnish with parsley to serve.

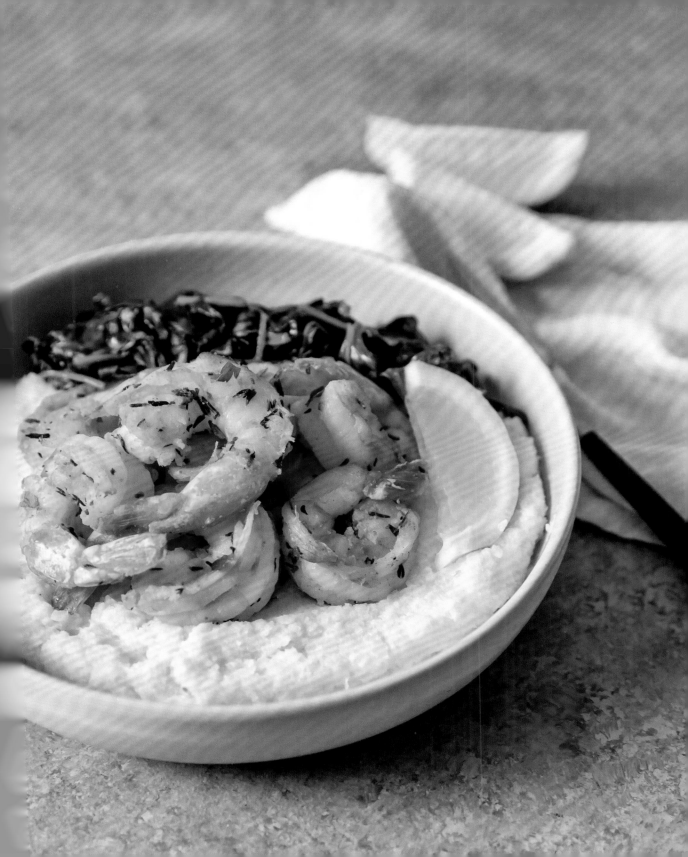

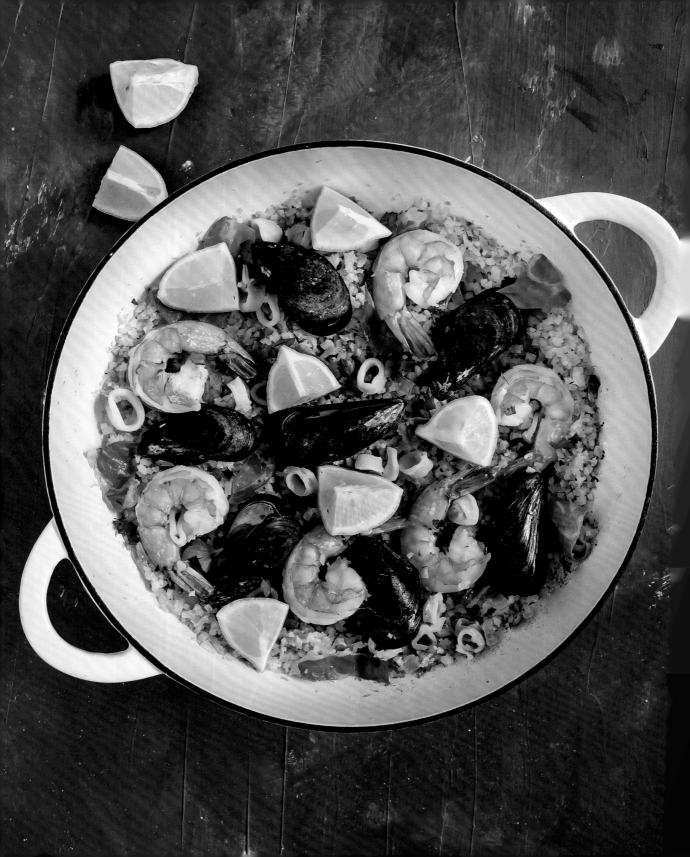

SEAFOOD AND PROSCIUTTO PAELLA

Paella is a Spanish dish often made with different types of seafood, saffron, paprika, and white rice that's crisped on the bottom. This version is nightshade free but with crispy prosciutto to add a smoky flavor. It's an amazing dish to impress dinner guests and satisfy a seafood craving.

PREP TIME 15 minutes   **COOK TIME** 25 minutes   **YIELD** Makes 4 servings

2 tablespoons (28 ml) avocado oil

½ onion, diced

3 garlic cloves, minced

4 prosciutto slices, roughly chopped

1 large head cauliflower, riced

1 teaspoon dried oregano

¾ teaspoon sea salt, plus more as needed

½ teaspoon saffron threads

8 ounces (225 g) medium shrimp, peeled and deveined

8 ounces (225 g) mussels, scrubbed and debearded, if needed

6 to 8 calamari tubes, sliced

1 tablespoon (4 g) chopped fresh parsley

1 lemon, quartered

1. In a large pan over medium heat, heat the avocado oil.

2. Add the onion and garlic and sauté for 5 to 6 minutes or until the onion is translucent.

3. Add the prosciutto and sauté for 1 to 2 minutes or until crispy. Using tongs, remove the prosciutto.

4. Add the cauliflower rice, oregano, salt, and saffron threads to the pan. Sauté for 5 to 7 minutes or until the cauliflower is cooked and slightly crisp.

5. Arrange the shrimp, mussels, and calamari on top of the cauliflower, discarding any mussels that have already opened. Reduce the heat to medium-low and cover the pan. Cook for 8 to 10 minutes. The mussels should open and the shrimp should be pink. Discard any mussels that have not opened.

6. Garnish with parsley, serve with the lemon for squeezing, and additional salt, if desired.

TUNA ZOODLE CASSEROLE

Your average tuna noodle casserole is made with canned soup, milk, peas, tons of butter, egg noodles, and bread crumbs. This isn't your average tuna noodle casserole! It's made with spiralized zucchini—to look just like egg noodles—for a vegetable-forward meal.

PREP TIME 15 minutes   **COOK TIME** 30 minutes   **YIELD** Makes 5 to 6 servings

1 tablespoon plus 1 teaspoon coconut oil (19 g), divided

1 medium white onion, diced

1 garlic clove, chopped

1 celery stalk, chopped

2 cups (475 ml) coconut milk

1 tablespoon and 2 teaspoons (15 g) arrowroot starch

3 medium zucchini, ends trimmed, spiralized

2 cans (5 ounce [140 g]) tuna, drained

¾ teaspoon sea salt

1 tablespoon (4 g) chopped fresh parsley

1. Preheat the oven to 350°F (180°C, or gas mark 4) and lightly grease a casserole dish with 1 teaspoon of coconut oil. Set aside.

2. In a skillet over medium heat, heat the remaining 1 tablespoon (14 g) of coconut oil.

3. Add the onion, garlic, and celery and sauté for 5 to 6 minutes or until the onion is translucent and the celery is slightly soft. Remove from the heat.

4. In a medium bowl, whisk the coconut milk with the arrowroot until the mixture thickens.

5. In the prepared casserole dish, combine the cooked vegetables, zucchini noodles, tuna, coconut milk mixture, and salt. Stir until well combined. Bake for 15 to 20 minutes or until the zucchini softens. Top with the parsley and serve.

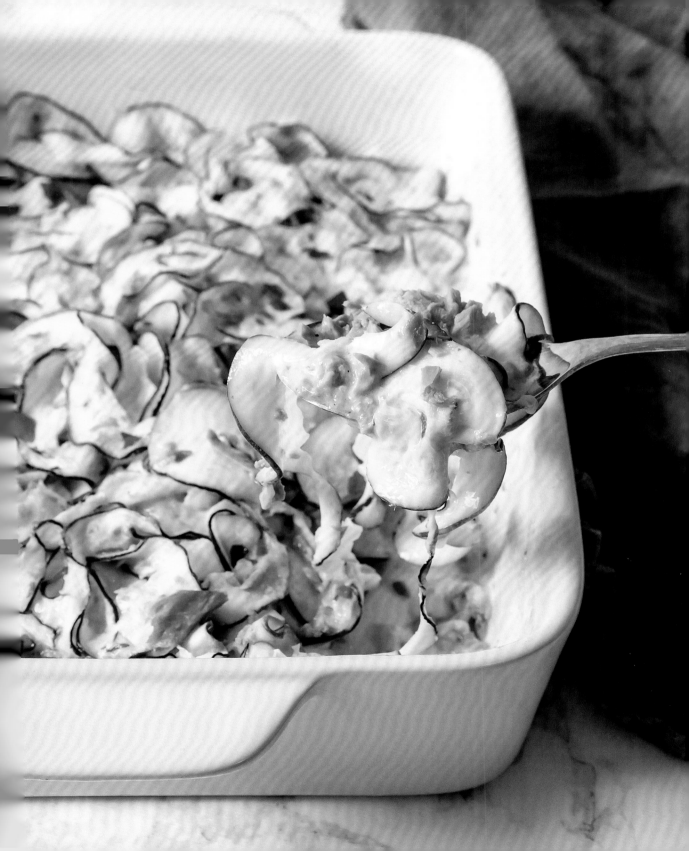

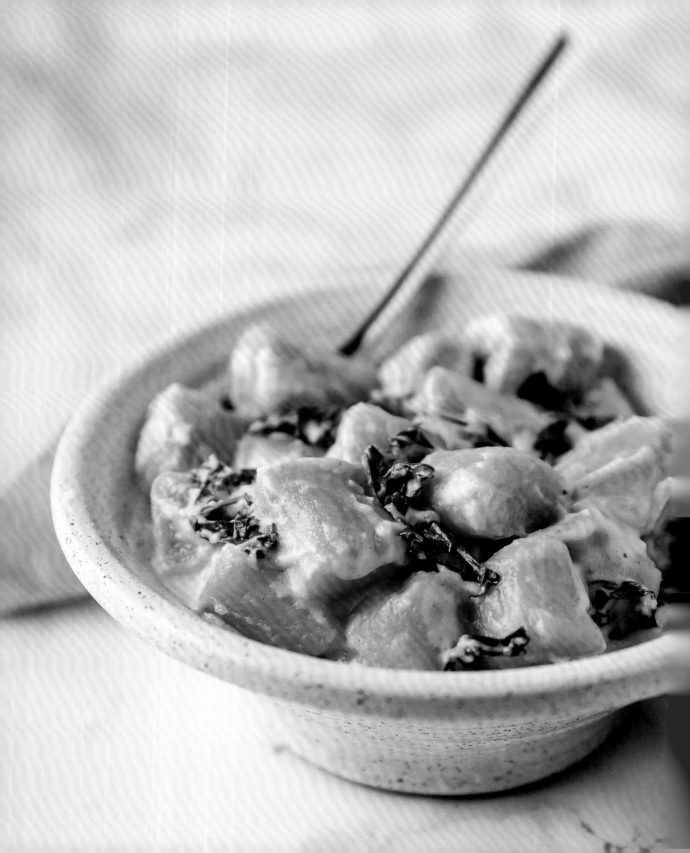

SWEET POTATO GNOCCHI WITH CREAM SAUCE

Gnocchi is an Italian dish that's traditionally made with white potato and flour. It's easily made AIP friendly with sweet potato, and it is the perfect pasta dish for when you're feeling a little fancy.

PREP TIME 20 minutes   **COOK TIME** 40 minutes   **YIELD** Makes 2 servings

FOR THE CREAM SAUCE

1 tablespoon (15 ml) olive oil

2 garlic cloves, minced

½ medium white onion, diced

1 cup (100 g) chopped cauliflower, steamed

½ cup (120 ml) coconut milk

¼ teaspoon sea salt

FOR THE GNOCCHI

1 cup (133 g) roughly chopped peeled sweet potato

⅓ cup (47 g) cassava flour

¼ cup (30 g) tapioca starch, plus more for dusting

6 tablespoons (90 ml) olive oil, divided

1 teaspoon sea salt

1 cup (67 g) chopped kale

1. To make the cream sauce: In a medium sauté pan or skillet over low heat, heat the olive oil.

2. Add the garlic and onion and sauté for 5 to 6 minutes or until the onion is translucent. Transfer to a high-speed blender.

3. Add the remaining sauce ingredients to the blender and blend until smooth. Set aside.

4. To make the gnocchi: In a medium pot, combine the sweet potato and enough water to cover. Place the pot over medium heat and bring to a low boil. Cook for 10 to 12 minutes or until the sweet potato is fork-tender. Drain the water and use a fork to mash the sweet potato. Set aside to cool.

5. In a large bowl, combine the cooled mashed sweet potato, cassava flour, tapioca starch, 1 tablespoon (15 ml) of olive oil, and salt. Knead until a dough forms.

6. Lightly dust a clean surface with tapioca starch. Turn out the dough onto the work surface. Divide it in half and roll each piece into a rope 6 to 8 inches (15 to 20 cm) long. Using a sharp knife, cut the ropes into small cylindrical gnocchi pieces, about 1 inch (2.5 cm) long.

7. Fill a medium pot about two-thirds full with water. Add 1 tablespoon (15 ml) of olive oil and the salt. Place the pot over high heat and bring to a boil. Add the gnocchi and boil until they float. Carefully strain the gnocchi in a colander. Drizzle with 1 tablespoon (15 ml) of olive oil to prevent them from sticking. Let cool.

8. In a medium sauté pan or skillet over medium-low heat, heat the remaining 1 tablespoon (15 ml) of olive oil.

9. Add the kale and stir until it wilts.

10. Add the gnocchi and sauté until lightly browned. Stir in the sauce and serve warm.

MARGHERITA PIZZA

As a native New Yorker, Italian by heritage, and self-proclaimed pizza enthusiast, I feel fully qualified to tell you this is the real deal. The crust holds up like traditional pizza crust, and the "cheese" is easily formed to look like real mozzarella. Now, *that's amore*!

PREP TIME 20 minutes   **COOK TIME** 40 minutes   **YIELD** 6 to 8 servings

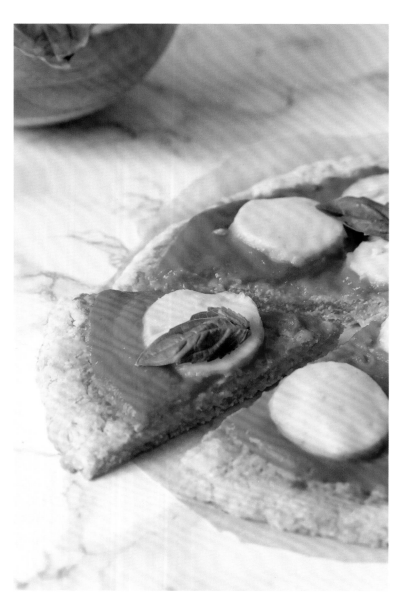

FOR THE "CHEESE"

1 ¼ cup (125 g) cauliflower, steamed

1 teaspoon lemon juice

2 tablespoons (28 ml) olive oil

1 tablespoon (15 ml) coconut milk

1 tablespoon (7 g) gelatin

1 tablespoon (4 g) nutritional yeast

1 tablespoon plus (7.5 g) tapioca starch

¼ teaspoon sea salt

FOR THE PIZZA

2 tablespoons plus 1 teaspoon (33 ml) olive oil

2 cups (200 g) cauliflower, riced

½ cup (64 g) arrowroot starch

¼ cup (28 g) coconut flour

2 tablespoons (8 g) nutritional yeast

¼ teaspoon baking soda

¼ teaspoon sea salt

1 teaspoon apple cider vinegar

1 Gelatin Egg (page 26)

¾ to 1 cup (188 to 250 g) Nightshade-Free "Tomato" Sauce (page 31)

Additional toppings, such as sliced black olives, sliced red onion, cooked chicken, cooked ground beef, prosciutto (optional)

Fresh basil leaves, for garnishing

1. To make the cauliflower "cheese:" While the cauliflower is still warm, use a nut milk bag, cheesecloth, or paper towel to carefully and lightly strain some, but not all, excess water from the steamed cauliflower. Transfer to a food processor.

2. Add the remaining "cheese" ingredients and blend until smooth. Spread the cheese mixture on the prepared plate into a flat layer about ½ inch (1 cm) thick. Freeze for 10 to 15 minutes to harden.

3. Add the remaining "cheese" ingredients and blend until smooth. Spread the cheese mixture on the prepared plate into a flat layer about ½ inch (1 cm) thick. Freeze for 15 to 20 minutes to harden.

4. Remove from the freezer and use a small circular mold (a measuring tablespoon works perfectly, but a small biscuit cutter or even a smooth bottle cap would work) to form small circular "cheese" pieces. Set aside in the refrigerator.

5. To make the pizza: Preheat the oven to 375°F (190°C). Line a baking sheet with parchment paper and lightly coat it with 1 teaspoon of olive oil.

6. In a medium pot, combine the riced cauliflower and enough water just to cover. Place the pot over medium heat and bring to a low simmer. Cover the pot and steam for about 7 minutes or until the cauliflower rice is soft. Drain the excess water from the pot and use a cheesecloth or nut milk bag to strain the cauliflower. You want the cauliflower to be fully strained and not holding any extra water.

7. In a large bowl, stir together the dry ingredients.

8. Fold in the riced cauliflower.

9. Stir in the remaining 2 tablespoons (28 ml) of olive oil and the vinegar.

10. Prepare the gelatin egg, add it to the cauliflower mixture, and mix until a dough forms. Press the dough onto the prepared baking sheet and form it into a thin circle, 8 to 9 inches (20 to 22 cm) in diameter. Bake for 15 to 18 minutes, or until the outer crust is lightly crisped

11. Top the crust with the "tomato" sauce and arrange the cauliflower "cheese" circles in an evenly spaced pattern. Add desired toppings (if using) and return to the oven for 5 to 7 minutes or until the toppings are warm.

12. Let cool slightly before slicing with a pizza cutter into 6 to 8 slices. Garnish with the basil.

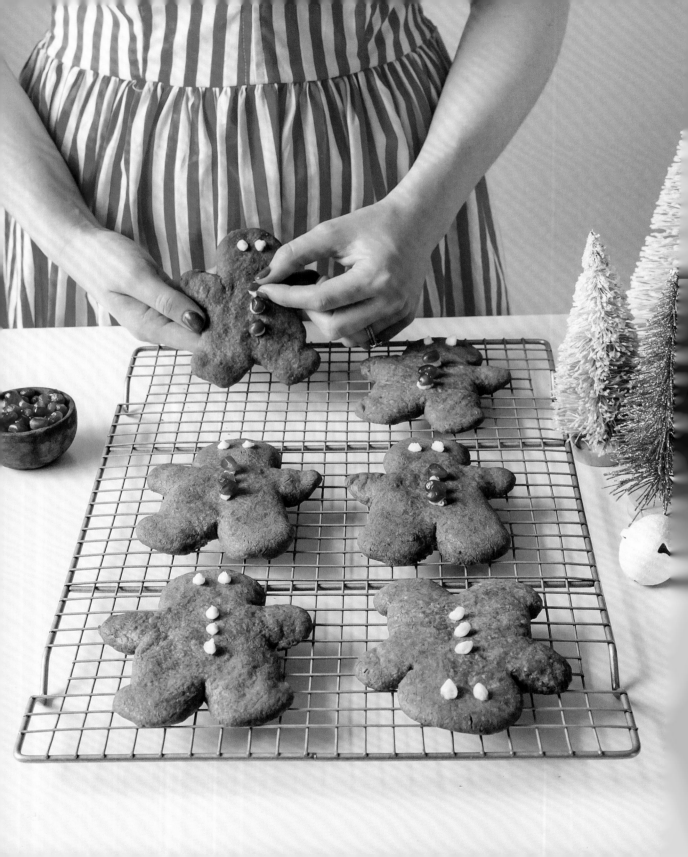

CHAPTER 7

HOLIDAY FAVORITES

The holidays are the time of year when you just want to kick back and indulge a little with loved ones. You don't want to have to worry about missing out on the comforting foods you love, but you also don't want to spoil your holiday eating food that makes you ill. It's a delicate balance that can often add more stress to an already stressful time of year.

You can have your gingerbread cookies and eat them, too! These holiday favorites are so good you'll be able to share with family and friends, and they won't be the wiser that they're all AIP!

← Gingerbread Cookies, page 167

ORANGE CRANBERRY SAUCE

I grew up eating cranberry sauce from a can. My dad loved it, and my mom would bring it to the Thanksgiving table *still* shaped like a can. It's not my favorite these days. This easy cranberry sauce is made without any refined sugar and has much more flavor than the stuff from the can! It's tart, sweet, and easy to make.

PREP TIME 5 minutes   **COOK TIME** 25 minutes   **YIELD** Makes 3 to 4 servings

3 cups (300 g) fresh cranberries

¾ cup (175 ml) fresh orange juice

⅓ cup (107 g) maple syrup

1 teaspoon ground cinnamon

Zest of ½ orange, divided

1. In a medium pot over medium heat, combine all the ingredients, reserving some of the orange zest for garnishing. Bring to a simmer and cook for 6 to 8 minutes until the cranberries start to pop. Continue to simmer, stirring occasionally, for 8 to 10 minutes more to reduce the liquid and until the bulk of the cranberries pop.

2. Remove from the heat and set aside to cool. Chill in the refrigerator. Serve topped with the remaining orange zest.

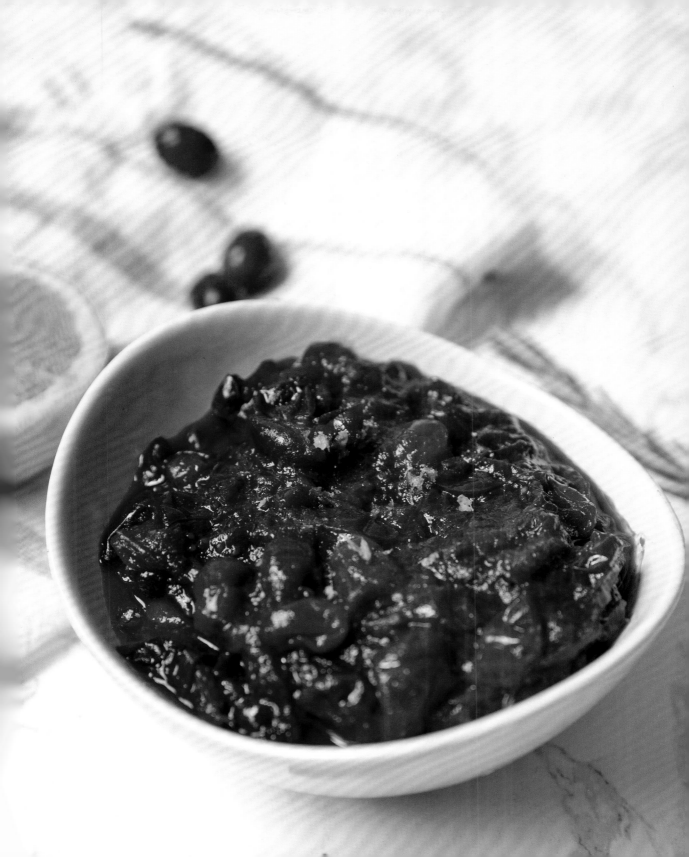

MUSHROOM GRAVY

Looking to sneak more vegetables onto your holiday table? This nutrient-dense mushroom gravy is just the thing!

PREP TIME 10 minutes   **COOK TIME** 25 minutes   **YIELD** Makes 3 to 4 servings

2 tablespoons (26 g) beef tallow

1 medium white onion, diced

1 garlic clove, minced

3 cups (210 g) chopped portobello mushrooms

1½ cups (355 ml) Chicken Bone Broth (page 25)

¼ teaspoon sea salt, plus more as needed

2 teaspoons fresh thyme leaves, chopped

2 to 3 teaspoons (6 to 9 g) arrowroot starch

1. In a medium saucepan over medium heat, melt the beef tallow.

2. Add the onion and garlic and sauté for 4 to 5 minutes, or until the onion is translucent.

3. Add the mushrooms and sauté for 4 to 5 minutes or until slightly softened.

4. Stir in the bone broth, salt, and thyme. Bring to a low simmer and cook for 5 to 10 minutes or until the mushrooms are fork-tender. Remove from the heat.

5. Let the gravy cool slightly before blending with an immersion blender or in a standard blender.

6. Return the pan to medium heat (and add the gravy if you've used a standard blender). Whisk in the arrowroot starch. Cook, whisking, until the gravy reaches the desired thickness. Taste, adjust the seasoning, and serve.

CAULIFLOWER STUFFING

PREP TIME 5 minutes   **COOK TIME** 30 minutes   **YIELD** Makes 4 servings

2 tablespoons (28 ml) avocado oil

1 yellow medium onion, diced

1 cup (70 g) diced mushrooms

1 cup (100 g) chopped celery

4 cups (400 g) cauliflower florets

¾ teaspoon sea salt, plus more as needed

1 tablespoon (2 g) fresh rosemary leaves, chopped

3 thyme sprigs, leaves removed

2 tablespoons (8 g) chopped fresh parsley

½ cup (120 ml) Chicken Bone Broth (page 25)

1. In a large deep skillet over medium heat, heat the avocado oil.

2. Add the onion and sauté for 5 to 6 minutes or until slightly translucent.

3. Add the mushrooms, celery, and cauliflower and cook for 6 to 7 minutes or until the vegetables are just fork-tender.

4. Stir in the salt, rosemary, thyme leaves, parsley, and bone broth. Cover the skillet, reduce the heat to medium-low, and simmer for 10 minutes or until most of the broth has reduced. Taste, adjust the seasoning, and serve.

ROASTED PARSNIP MASH

Missing mashed potatoes at the holidays? Look no further! Parsnips are a great potato substitute as they have a similar texture and help mix it up when you want something else other than sweet potatoes. You can just as easily boil parsnips to make a mash, but roasting them brings out so much more flavor and texture!

PREP TIME 10 minutes   **COOK TIME** 25 minutes   **YIELD** Makes 3 to 4 servings

4 cups (440 g) chopped peeled parsnip

2 garlic cloves, peeled and smashed

4 tablespoons (60 ml) avocado oil, divided

2 thyme sprigs, leaves removed

2 tablespoons (4 g) fresh rosemary leaves, chopped

¾ teaspoon sea salt, plus more as needed

1 cup (235 ml) coconut milk

1. Preheat the oven to 400°F (200°C, or gas mark 6) and line a baking sheet with parchment paper.

2. Place the parsnip and garlic on the prepared baking sheet. Add 2 tablespoons (28 ml) of the avocado oil and toss to coat evenly. Spread them out and sprinkle with the thyme, rosemary, and salt. Bake for 25 minutes, or until the parsnips are fork-tender and slightly crisp.

3. Let cool slightly before transferring to a food processor.

4. Add the remaining 2 tablespoons (28 ml) of avocado oil and the coconut milk. Blend until smooth and no large chunks remain. Taste, adjust the seasoning, and serve.

SWEET POTATO LATKES

It doesn't feel like Hanukkah without latkes! I grew up in a half-Jewish, half-Catholic home, and I loved when my mom made latkes. Latkes are traditionally made with white potatoes, but sweet potatoes are a heathier and sweeter alternative. I like to use white Hannah sweet potatoes when possible, but orange potatoes work, too.

PREP TIME 15 minutes   **COOK TIME** 25 minutes   **YIELD** Makes 3 to 4 servings

2 cups (300 g) shredded sweet potato, (see Notes)

½ white onion, finely diced

¼ cup (28 g) coconut flour

¼ cup (30 g) tapioca starch

½ teaspoon sea salt

¼ cup plus 2 tablespoons (84 g) coconut oil, plus more as needed

Coconut Yogurt (page 37), for serving

Applesauce, for serving

1. Line a plate with paper towels and set aside.

2. In a large bowl, combine the sweet potato, onion, coconut flour, tapioca starch, salt, and 2 tablespoons (28 g) of coconut oil. Mix until thoroughly combined.

3. In a large deep skillet over medium heat, heat the remaining ¼ cup (55 g) of coconut oil.

4. Form the sweet potato mixture into patties the size of your palm and lightly flatten them. You want the latkes ¼ to ⅓ inch (6 to 8 mm) thick. You should have about 4 to 5 latkes.

5. One or two at a time, carefully drop the latkes into the hot oil. Cook for 3 to 4 minutes on each side or until golden brown, carefully flipping with a spatula. Transfer the cooked latkes to the prepared plate. Repeat with the remaining latkes, adding more oil as needed.

6. Serve with coconut yogurt and applesauce on the side.

NOTES

I find it best to use a box cheese grater to grate the sweet potato to get the classic latke look and texture.

BACON CHIVE "CORN" BREAD

"Corn" bread is a bit of a misnomer when it doesn't actually have any corn in it. However, this tastes like real corn bread! With corn bread's classic texture and some savory add-ins such as the bacon and chives, this is an amazing addition to your holiday table or the perfect side with Butternut Bison Chili (page 77).

PREP TIME 25 minutes   **COOK TIME** 20 minutes   **YIELD** Makes 9 servings

Coconut oil, for preparing the pan

1 cup (112 g) coconut flour

¼ cup plus 2 tablespoons (54 g) arrowroot starch

½ teaspoon baking soda

3 cooked bacon slices, chopped and patted dry

1 tablespoon (3 g) chopped fresh chives

¼ teaspoon sea salt

3 tablespoons (39 g) palm shortening

2 tablespoons (40 g) honey, plus more for serving

½ cup (120 ml) coconut milk

1 teaspoon apple cider vinegar

3 Gelatin Eggs (page 26, see Notes)

1. Preheat the oven to 350°F (180°C, or gas mark 4). Line an 8 × 8-inch (20 x 20 cm) baking pan with parchment paper and lightly coat it with coconut oil. Set aside.

2. In a large bowl, stir together the coconut flour, arrowroot starch, baking soda, bacon, chives, and salt.

3. Add the palm shortening and honey and stir until well combined.

4. In a medium bowl, stir together the coconut milk and vinegar. Pour the mixture into the corn bread dough and stir to combine.

5. Prepare the gelatin eggs and add them to the dough. Stir to combine. Spoon the dough into the prepared baking pan and evenly spread with the back of a spoon or a rubber spatula. Bake for 20 minutes or until the top is lightly golden brown.

6. Carefully remove the corn bread from the pan using the parchment and transfer to a cooling rack. Let cool completely before slicing. The bread needs to set or it will be gummy if you slice it too early.

7. Cut into nine pieces and enjoy topped with honey.

NOTES

For the three gelatin eggs, triple the recipe and make them all in one batch rather than making individual gelatin eggs. Use immediately.

ROAST CHICKEN

This roast chicken is simple and flavorful. It's a great addition to a holiday table, or, really, enjoyed any day of the year.

PREP TIME 10 minutes   **COOK TIME** 1 hour   **YIELD** Makes 3 to 4 servings

1 (5 to 6 pounds [2.23 to 2.7 kg]) whole chicken

1 lemon, halved

3 tablespoons (45 ml) avocado oil

5 garlic cloves, finely minced

2 tablespoons (4 g) fresh rosemary leaves, chopped

2 teaspoons fresh thyme leaves, chopped

½ teaspoon sea salt

1 medium onion, quartered

1. Preheat the oven to 400°F (200°C, or gas mark 6).

2. Pat the chicken dry and place it in a large roasting pan.

3. Squeeze the juice from one lemon half into a small bowl. Add the avocado oil, garlic, rosemary, thyme, and salt and whisk to combine.

4. Quarter the other lemon half and place the pieces inside the chicken's cavity along with the onion.

5. Use a knife to carefully separate the chicken skin from the chicken without removing it. Spoon 1 tablespoon of the oil mixture under the skin. Pour the remainder of the oil mixture over the chicken and use your hands to generously coat. Bake for 1 hour, or until the internal temperature reaches 165°F (74°C) on a meat thermometer inserted into the thigh.

6. Let the chicken rest for 15 to 20 minutes. Remove the onion and lemon from the cavity before slicing and serving.

GINGERBREAD COOKIES

Make amazing memories and yummy treats at the same time with these cute little gingerbread cookies! These cookies are fun to make and decorate with loved ones and even more fun to eat. They're charming—with their frosting eyes and pomegranate buttons—but you can get creative with more toppings and decorations.

PREP TIME 25 minutes **COOK TIME** 12 minutes **YIELD** Makes 5 to 6 servings

FOR THE COOKIES

Coconut oil, for preparing the baking sheet

¾ cup (90 g) tapioca starch

½ cup (56 g) tigernut flour

1 tablespoon (7 g) gelatin

½ teaspoon baking soda

1 teaspoon ground ginger

½ teaspoon ground cinnamon

⅓ cup (69 g) palm shortening

3 tablespoons (60 g) maple syrup

2 tablespoons (40 g) blackstrap molasses

½ teaspoon vanilla extract

FOR THE FROSTING AND DECORATIONS

¼ cup (52 g) palm shortening

1 tablespoon (20 g) light-colored honey

1 to 2 tablespoons (11 to 22 g) pomegranate seeds

1. To make the cookies: Preheat the oven to 350°F (180°C, or gas mark 4). Line a baking sheet with parchment paper and lightly coat it with coconut oil. Set aside.

2. In a large bowl, combine the dry ingredients.

3. In a medium bowl, cream together the palm shortening, maple syrup, and molasses. Add the wet mixture to the dry ingredients. Stir in the vanilla extract and combine well until all ingredients are blended and form a dough. Transfer the dough to a pastry board or clean piece of parchment.

4. Working with about ½ cup (about 65 g) of dough at a time, flatten it to about ¼ inch (6 mm) thick. Use a gingerbread cookie cutter to cut the dough and pull away from the excess dough around the cookie cutter with your fingers. Return any excess dough to the bowl. Transfer the formed gingerbread cookies onto the prepared baking sheet. Repeat the process with the remainder of the dough, evenly spacing the cookies on the baking sheet. You should have five to six cookies. Bake for 10 to 12 minutes or until the cookies are a light golden brown.

5. Carefully transfer to a cooling rack and let cool completely before decorating.

6. To make the frosting and decorations: In a medium bowl, cream together the palm shortening and honey and transfer to a piping bag. Pipe eyes and other features onto the gingerbread people. Use pomegranate seeds for buttons. Enjoy!

CRANBERRY CHEESECAKE BARS

Cheesecake without any cheese? Yes! These cranberry cheesecake bars are creamy, tart, and perfect for a fun Christmas dessert.

PREP TIME 3 hour, 10 minutes   **COOK TIME** 10 minutes   **YIELD** Makes 9 servings

FOR THE CRUST

10 pitted dates

1 cup (80 g) shredded unsweetened coconut

1 tablespoon (14 g) coconut oil

FOR THE FILLING

1½ cups (355 g) coconut cream

2 tablespoons (28 g) coconut oil

¼ cup (80 g) honey

1 tablespoon (15 ml) fresh orange juice

Zest of ½ orange

⅛ teaspoon sea salt

1 tablespoon (7 g) gelatin

FOR THE CRANBERRY TOPPING

2 cups (200 g) whole cranberries

⅓ cup (80 ml) fresh orange juice

¼ cup (80 g) maple syrup

Zest of ½ orange

1. To make the crust: Line the bottom of an 8 x 8-inch (20 x 20 cm) baking pan with parchment paper and set aside.

2. If the dates are hard, soak them in enough warm water to cover for 5 minutes or until they soften. Drain. Blend the dates in a food processor. Add the coconut and coconut oil and blend until fully combined. Evenly press the crust mixture onto the bottom of the prepared pan and set aside.

3. To make the filling: In a medium pot over low heat, combine the coconut cream, coconut oil, and honey. Cook, stirring, until the mixture melts and is fully incorporated. Remove from heat and stir in the orange juice, zest, and salt.

4. Sprinkle the gelatin into the pot and whisk until it is fully combined and melted. Pour the filling into the prepared pan over the crust and refrigerate to harden for 3 to 4 hours or overnight.

5. To make the cranberry topping: In a small saucepan over medium heat, combine the cranberry topping ingredients. Bring to a simmer. Cook for about 8 minutes, stirring, until the majority of cranberries pop and the sauce thickens and reduces. Remove from the heat and let cool.

6. Remove the bars from the refrigerator, cut into nine slices, and top each with cranberry topping.

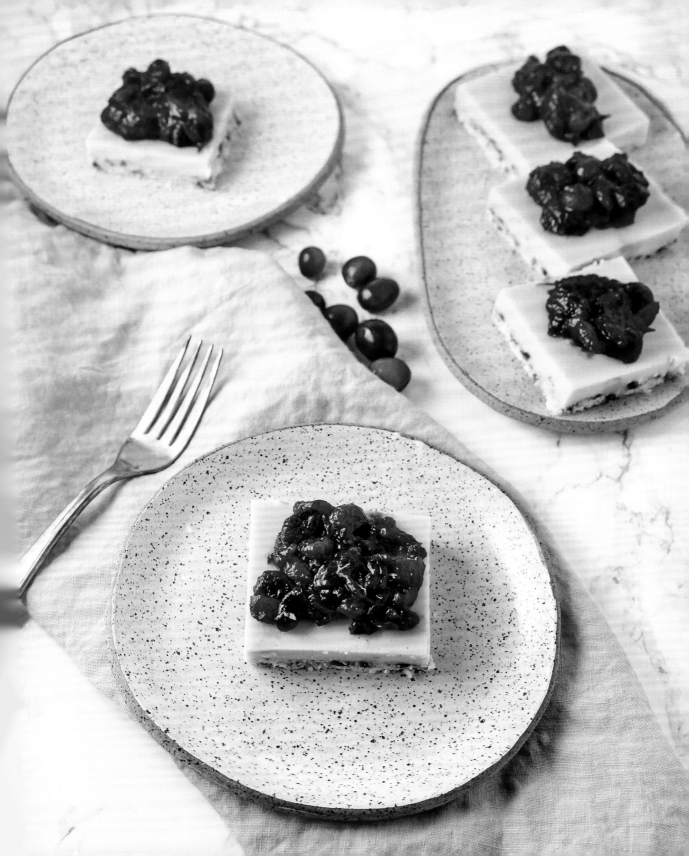

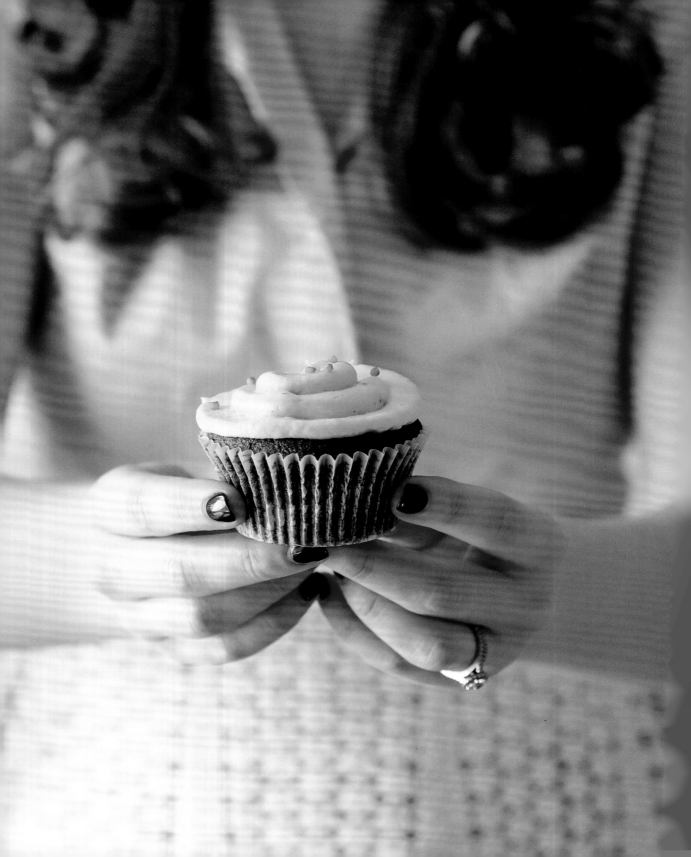

CHAPTER 8

DECADENT DESSERTS & DRINKS

If you feel as though starting the AIP means you can no longer enjoy a fun treat, think again! I've got you covered in this chapter. Look forward to cookies, scones, cupcakes, brownies, and more.

Remember the core of the AIP is healing, nutrient-dense food. However, life goes on and sometimes you just need a cupcake on your birthday. Moderation is key, but you don't have to kiss desserts good-bye forever!

← "Chocolate" Birthday Cupcakes with Pomegranate Frosting, page 180

COFFEE SHOP PUMPKIN SCONES

Throw on your favorite flannel, scarf, and riding boots! These pumpkin scones are the perfect copycat for those you'd find as a seasonal treat in a local café or coffee shop. They're perfect for a post-pumpkin–picking treat, part of a brisk autumn brunch, or for getting fancy at a Halloween party.

PREP TIME 15 minutes   **COOK TIME** 25 minutes   **YIELD** Makes 6 scones

¼ cup (56 g) coconut oil, plus more for preparing the baking sheet

1¼ cups (140 g) tigernut flour

3 tablespoons (21 g) coconut flour

¼ cup (30 g) tapioca starch

1 teaspoon ground cinnamon, plus more for garnishing

¼ teaspoon baking soda

¼ cup (80 g) maple syrup

3 tablespoons (46 g) pumpkin purée

1 Gelatin Egg (page 26)

2 tablespoons (28 g) coconut butter, melted (see Notes)

1 tablespoon (14 g) coconut oil, melted

1 teaspoon honey

1. Preheat the oven to 350°F (180°C, or gas mark 4). Line a baking sheet with parchment paper and lightly coat it with coconut oil.

2. In a medium bowl, sift together the tigernut and coconut flours, tapioca starch, cinnamon, and baking soda.

3. Stir in the coconut oil, maple syrup, and pumpkin purée.

4. Prepare the Gelatin Egg and add it to the dough. Mix well to combine and form into a dough. Place the dough on a cutting board and form it into a large circle, about 1 inch (2.5 cm) thick. Use a pizza cutter or knife to slice the dough into six triangular scones. Place them on the prepared baking sheet and bake for 20 to 25 minutes or until fully cooked.

5. Transfer to a cooling rack to cool completely.

6. In a small bowl, whisk the melted coconut butter, coconut oil, and honey. Drizzle the icing over the scones and sprinkle with cinnamon.

NOTES

The preferred method for melting coconut butter is using a double boiler (see Glazed "Chocolate" Doughnut Holes, page 175).

If the icing is too thick, add more coconut oil.

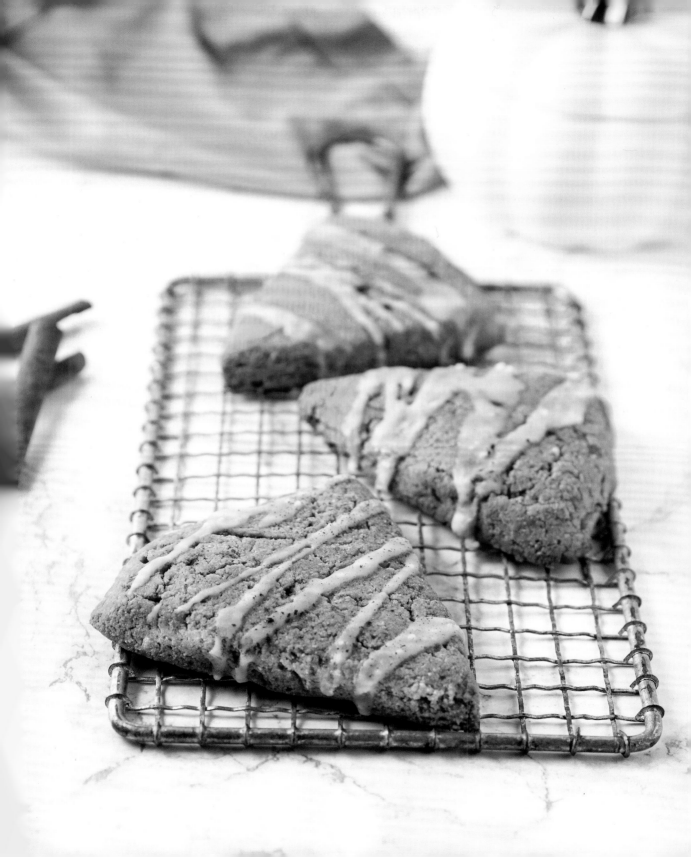

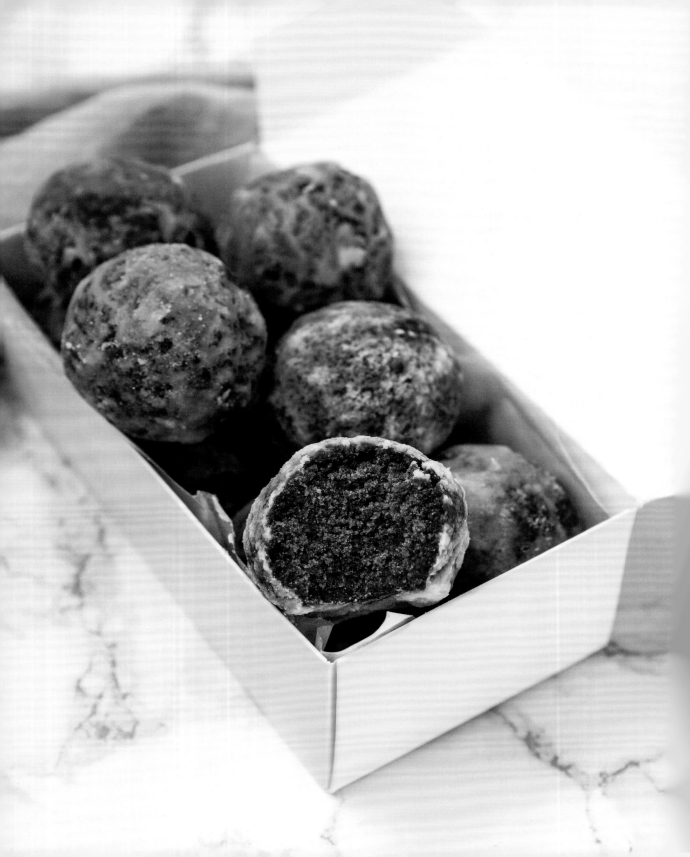

GLAZED "CHOCOLATE" DOUGHNUT HOLES

Glazed chocolate cake doughnut holes were my favorite treat to get at our local doughnut shop when I was a kid. When I went gluten free, I was constantly searching for the perfect substitute. This recipe is the closest thing to the real deal! It's cakey, it holds together, and it's so simple to make!

PREP TIME 15 minutes   **COOK TIME** 12 minutes   **YIELD** Makes 8 to 9 doughnut holes

⅓ cup (37 g) tigernut flour

¼ cup (28 g) coconut flour

¼ cup (30 g) tapioca starch

2 tablespoons (16 g) carob powder

1 tablespoon (7 g) gelatin

¼ teaspoon baking soda

¼ cup (80 g) maple syrup

⅓ cup (69 g) palm shortening

3 tablespoons (39 g) coconut butter

¼ cup (56 g) coconut oil

2 teaspoons light-colored honey

1. Preheat the oven to 350°F (180°C, or gas mark 4) and line a baking sheet with parchment paper. Set aside.

2. In a medium bowl, stir together the tigernut and coconut flours, tapioca starch, carob powder, gelatin, and baking soda until fully combined.

3. Pour in the maple syrup and lightly mix. Fold in the palm shortening until the mixture is creamy. Form the dough into eight or nine doughnut holes and place them on the prepared baking sheet. Bake for 10 to 12 minutes or until the doughnut holes are hardened on the outside. Remove and let cool to the touch.

4. Assemble a double boiler with a medium pot filled halfway with water and bring the water to a simmer over low heat. Place a metal mixing bowl over the pot. Add the coconut butter and coconut oil to the bowl and let it slowly melt, stirring often. Once completely melted, use an oven mitt to remove the bowl from the heat.

5. Whisk in the honey until well combined.

6. Dip the doughnut holes in the glaze several times until completely coated and place on a plate. Refrigerate for 15 to 20 minutes to harden the glaze.

NOTES

The best way to melt coconut butter is a double boiler method described here. Avoid using the microwave as it will burn the coconut butter.

"CHOCOLATE" CHUNK COOKIES

It's not a comfort food cookbook without chocolate chip cookies. As my all-time favorite dessert, I've spent hours perfecting the tastiest AIP-compliant cookie. These are *it*! Chocolate is out during the AIP elimination phase, so these cookies are made with homemade carob chips.

PREP TIME 10 minutes   **COOK TIME** 40 minutes   **YIELD** Makes 9 or 10 cookies

FOR THE CAROB CHUNKS

¾ cup (156 g) coconut butter

¼ cup (56 g) coconut oil

¼ cup (32 g) carob powder

3 tablespoons (60 g) maple syrup

FOR THE COOKIES

1 cup (112 g) tigernut flour

¼ cup (30 g) tapioca starch

1 tablespoon (7 g) gelatin

⅛ teaspoon baking soda

⅛ teaspoon sea salt

¼ cup (80 g) maple syrup

⅓ cup (75 g) coconut oil

½ teaspoon vanilla extract

3 tablespoons (23 g) Carob Chunks (recipe follows)

1. To make the carob chunks: Assemble a double boiler with a medium pot filled halfway with water and bring the water to a simmer over low heat. Place a metal mixing bowl over the pot. Add the coconut butter and coconut oil to the bowl and let it slowly melt, stirring often. Once completely melted, use an oven mitt to remove the bowl from the heat.

2. Using a fine-mesh sifter, sift the carob powder into the mixture to ensure there are no clumps. Stir to mix and then stir in the maple syrup until thoroughly combined. Pour the mixture into a mold. (I use a small, heat-resistant glass container, but a silicone mold would also work.) Let cool slightly before placing in the freezer for 20 to 25 minutes. Chop the carob into small chunks. Return to the freezer for about 1 hour or until fully hardened.

3. To make the cookies: Preheat the oven to 375°F (190°C, or gas mark 5) and line a baking sheet with parchment paper. Set aside.

4. In a medium bowl, sift together the tigernut flour, tapioca starch, gelatin, baking soda, and salt.

5. Stir in the maple syrup, coconut oil, and vanilla until thoroughly combined. Fold in the carob chunks. Divide the batter into nine or ten pieces, roll each into a ball, and place on the prepared baking sheet, evenly spaced. Slightly flatten each with the palm of your hand. Bake for 10 to 12 minutes. Transfer to a wire rack to cool for 15 to 20 minutes before enjoying.

NOTES

You'll have leftover carob chunks. Refrigerate them for about one week or freeze for about one month. Eat them for snacks or use in the Mint Chip Brownies (page 179).

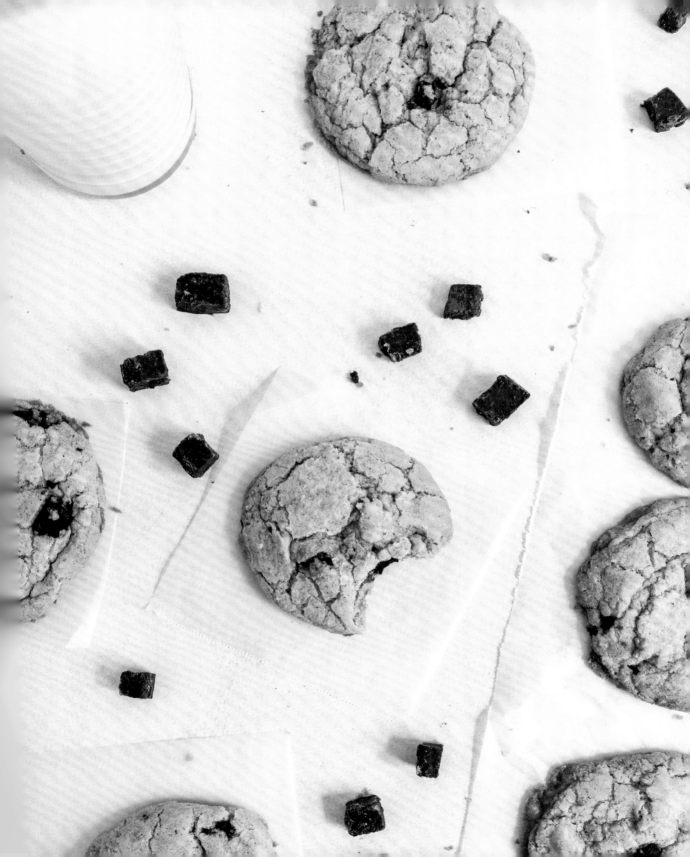

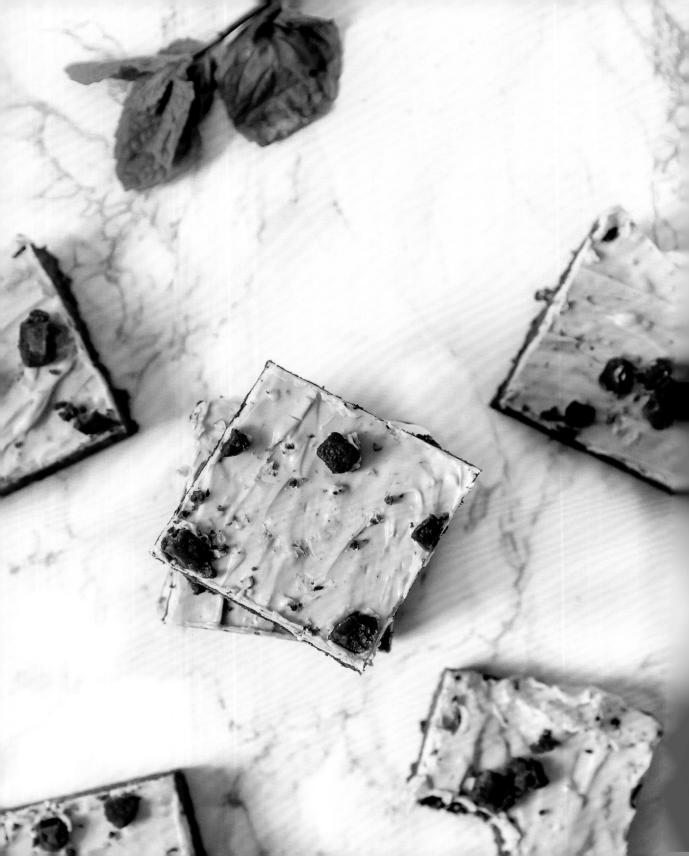

MINT CHIP BROWNIES

There's nothing like the smell and taste of fresh mint, especially when it's paired with rich brownies and a creamy frosting. These brownies are heavy on the mint flavor and are an all-around decadent and fun treat.

PREP TIME 25 minutes   **COOK TIME** 30 minutes   **YIELD** Makes 9 brownies

FOR THE BROWNIES

⅓ cup (75 g) coconut oil, plus more for preparing the baking pan

1 cup (112 g) tigernut flour

¼ cup (30 g) tapioca starch

3 tablespoons (24 g) carob powder

¼ teaspoon baking soda

⅛ teaspoon sea salt

⅓ cup (107 g) maple syrup

1 Gelatin Egg (page 26)

¼ to ⅓ cup (30 to 40 g) carob chunks (see "Chocolate" Chunk Cookies, page 176)

FOR THE MINT FROSTING

½ cup (104 g) palm shortening

½ cup (120 g) coconut cream

¼ to ½ teaspoon matcha powder (adjust for desired color)

2 tablespoons (40 g) maple syrup

1 tablespoon (6 g) fresh mint leaves, chopped

1. To make the brownies: Preheat the oven to 350°F (180°C). Line an 8 x 8-inch (20 x 20 cm) baking pan with parchment paper and lightly coat it with coconut oil. Set aside.

2. In a large bowl, stir together the dry ingredients.

3. Add the coconut oil and maple syrup and stir to combine.

4. Prepare the gelatin egg and stir it into the batter until fully combined. Pour the batter into the prepared baking pan, spreading it evenly with the back of a spoon. Bake for 25 minutes or until done—when a toothpick inserted into the center comes out clean.

5. Let cool slightly and then lift the parchment paper to help transfer the brownies to a wire rack to cool completely.

6. To make the mint frosting: In a food processor, combine the palm shortening, coconut cream, matcha powder, maple syrup, and mint. Process until there are no large pieces of mint left. The color should be light green. Using a rubber spatula, evenly spread the topping over the brownies. Refrigerate for 10 to 15 minutes to set.

7. Chop the carob chunks into small pieces and sprinkle over the brownies. Cut into nine pieces and serve chilled.

NOTES

The mint frosting will melt a little if the brownies are left out too long. Keep them chilled!

"CHOCOLATE" BIRTHDAY CUPCAKES WITH POMEGRANATE FROSTING

Nothing replaces cake on your birthday! When I first started dealing with autoimmune disease and food intolerances and my birthday rolled around, my birthday cake was nothing short of bizarre and, honestly, not very tasty. Not these cupcakes! These birthday cupcakes have the *perfect* texture and are topped with a traditional frosting—with sprinkles!

PREP TIME 60 minutes   **COOK TIME** 25 minutes   **YIELD** Makes 6 cupcakes

FOR THE CUPCAKES

1 cup (121 g) tigernut flour

¼ cup (30 g) tapioca starch

3 tablespoons (24 g) carob powder

¼ teaspoon baking soda

½ cup (112 g) coconut oil, melted

¼ cup (80 g) maple syrup

1 Gelatin Egg (page 26)

FOR THE SPRINKLES

2 tablespoons (22 g) tapioca pearls

2 tablespoons (28 ml) pomegranate juice

FOR THE FROSTING

⅔ cup (139 g) palm shortening

2 teaspoons light-colored honey

2 tablespoons (15 g) tapioca starch

1 to 2 teaspoons pomegranate juice

1. To make the cupcakes: Preheat the oven to 350°F (180°C, or gas mark 4) and line a muffin tin with six cupcake liners. Set aside.

2. In a large bowl, stir together the tigernut flour, tapioca starch, carob powder, and baking soda.

3. Add the melted coconut oil and maple syrup and stir to combine.

4. Prepare the gelatin egg, add to the mixture, mixing well to form a batter. Spoon the batter into the cupcake liners until two-thirds full. Bake for 23 to 25 minutes, or until baked through—when a toothpick inserted into the center comes out clean.

5. Carefully transfer the cupcakes to a cooling rack and allow to come to room temperature before allowing to cool further and set in the refrigerator for 20 to 30 minutes.

6. To make the sprinkles: While the cupcakes cool, combine the tapioca pearls and pomegranate juice in a small bowl. Set aside for 20 to 30 minutes while the tapioca pearls soften and absorb the pomegranate juice.

7. To make the frosting: In a medium bowl, cream together the palm shortening, honey, and tapioca starch until smooth.

8. One teaspoon at a time, stir in the pomegranate juice until the frosting reaches the desired color. Set aside in a cool place.

9. Top the prepared cupcakes with frosting and sprinkles.

NOTES

Carefully transfer the cupcakes to a cooling rack and allow to come to room temperature before allowing to cool further and set in the refrigerator for 20 to 30 minutes before topping with the frosting and sprinkles.

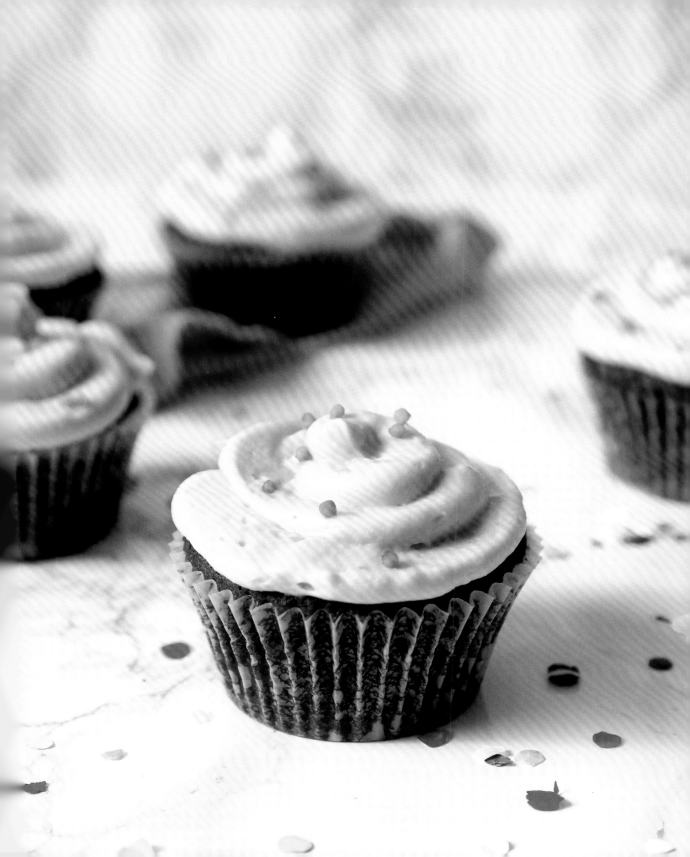

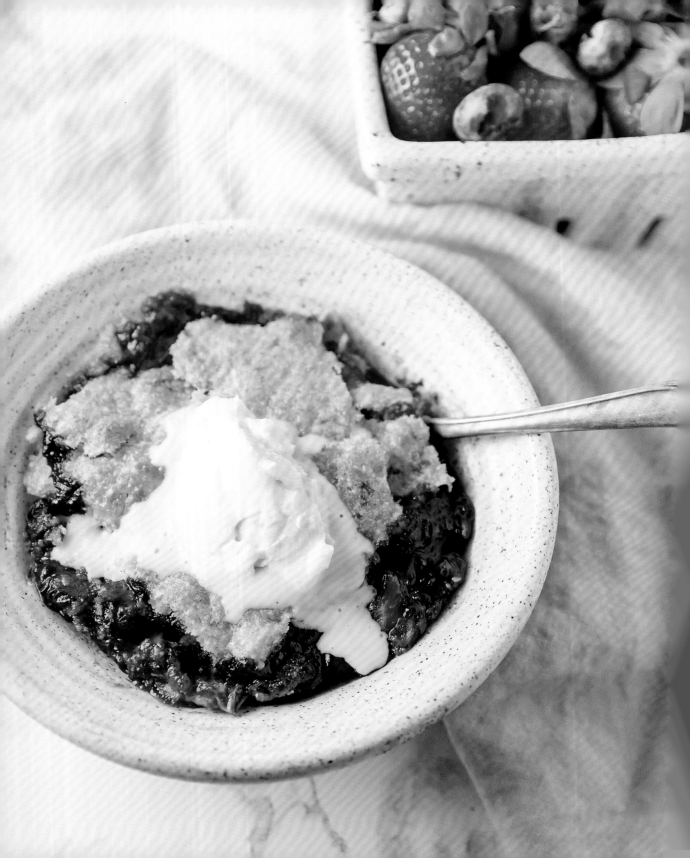

SUMMER BERRY CRISP

This crisp is made for summer! The mix of tangy and sweet is perfectly refreshing on a hot summer day or as a light dessert after dinner. The crispy and crumbly topping provides just the right amount of crunch. If you're looking to really indulge or impress guests, I recommend topping it with coconut cream or homemade AIP-compliant coconut ice cream for an even more decadent treat.

PREP TIME 15 minutes   **COOK TIME** 40 minutes   **YIELD** Makes 5 to 6 servings

FOR THE FILLING

4 cups (580 g) fresh strawberries, quartered

1 cup (145 g) fresh blueberries

2 tablespoons (18 g) arrowroot starch

2 teaspoons fresh lemon juice

FOR THE TOPPING

¾ cup (60 g) shredded unsweetened coconut

⅓ cup (37 g) tigernut flour

¼ cup (36 g) arrowroot starch

1 tablespoon (7 g) coconut flour

½ teaspoon ground cinnamon

⅛ teaspoon sea salt

¼ cup (56 g) coconut oil

¼ cup (80 g) maple syrup

½ cup (120 g) coconut cream (optional)

1. Preheat the oven to 375°F (190°C, or gas mark 5).

2. To make the filling: In an 8 x 8-inch (20 x 20 cm) baking dish, combine the filling ingredients and mix well. Set aside.

3. To make the topping: In a large bowl, stir together the dry ingredients.

4. Add the wet ingredients and stir until a dough forms. Use your hands to press the dough over the top of the filling to cover it. Bake for 35 to 40 minutes or until the topping has crisped and browned.

5. Let cool before serving with coconut cream, if desired.

SOUTHERN FRIED APPLES

These apples are the perfect solution when you want something sweet but don't want to bake. They are more tart than sweet, yet still satisfy a craving.

PREP TIME 10 minutes   **COOK TIME** 8 minutes   **YIELD** Makes 4 servings

4 Granny Smith apples, peeled, cored, and sliced

2 tablespoons (18 g) coconut sugar

1 teaspoon ground cinnamon

1 tablespoon (15 ml) fresh lemon juice

2 tablespoons (28 g) coconut oil

1. In a large bowl, combine the apples, coconut sugar, cinnamon, and lemon juice. Using your hands, mix until the apples are thoroughly coated.

2. In a large deep skillet over medium-low heat, melt the coconut oil.

3. Add the apples. Cook for 6 to 8 minutes or until the apples are soft and the sugar has dissolved. Serve warm.

ORANGE TURMERIC GUMMIES

Gummy bears, surprisingly, don't have to be unhealthy. These homemade gummies have two health-promoting secret ingredients—gelatin and turmeric! Make these as a nostalgic snack or a simple immunity booster.

PREP TIME 115 minutes, plus 2 hours chilling time   **COOK TIME** Cook time: 15 minutes   **YIELD** Varies depending on the mold used

1 cup (235 ml) fresh orange juice

1 cup (175 g) chopped mango

¼ cup (28 g) gelatin

2 tablespoons (40 g) honey

2 teaspoons ground turmeric

1. In a high-speed blender, combine the orange juice and mango. Blend until liquefied. Transfer to a large pot over medium-low heat.

2. Whisk in the gelatin, honey, and turmeric until it thickens. Cook for 10 minutes, whisking occasionally, or until the mixture becomes a thin liquid. Pour the mixture into a silicone gummy mold or heatproof glass dish. Let cool slightly before refrigerating for at least 2 hours. Slice and serve chilled.

FRUITY SANGRIA

Sangria is a refreshing drink made with Spanish wine, citrus fruit, and apples. This mocktail version is just as tasty! Serve it at a summer picnic or cookout to cool off on a warm day.

PREP TIME 15 minutes   **YIELD** Makes 5 servings

1 Granny Smith apple, washed well, cored, and thinly sliced

1 medium orange, washed well, thinly sliced, and seeded

1 lime, washed well and thinly sliced

½ lemon, washed well, thinly sliced, and seeded

2 cups (475 ml) 100% no-sugar-added grape juice

2 cups (475 ml) sparkling water

½ cup (120 ml) fresh orange juice

In a large pitcher, combine the apple, orange, lime, and lemon slices. Pour in the grape juice, sparkling water, and orange juice. Stir well to combine. Serve chilled.

FROZEN GRAPEFRUIT MARGARITA

Hold the tequila and keep all the flavor and fun with this festive mocktail! Serve this easy drink on Cinco de Mayo, or for a fun night in.

PREP TIME 5 minutes   **YIELD** Makes 2 servings

1 teaspoon sea salt

1 to 2 lime wedges, plus more for garnishing

2½ cups (250 g) crushed ice

1 cup (235 ml) fresh grapefruit juice

¼ cup (60 ml) fresh lime juice

2 tablespoons (40 g) honey

2 to 3 slices fresh grapefruit (optional)

1. Place the salt on a small plate. Run a lime wedge around the rims of two glasses and dip them in the salt. Shake off the excess and set aside.

2. In a high-speed blender, combine the ice, grapefruit and lime juices, and honey. Blend until mixed. Pour the margarita into the prepared glasses and serve garnished with lime wedges or grapefruit slices.

HOT COCOA

There's nothing like a mug of hot cocoa on a cold winter's day. Serve this hot cocoa to warm up or as a sweet treat.

PREP TIME 5 minutes   **COOK TIME** 10 minutes   **YIELD** Makes 2 servings

2 cups (475 ml) coconut milk (see Apple Cinnamon Granola with Coconut Milk, page 38), or canned coconut milk

2 tablespoons (30 g) coconut cream, plus more for serving (optional)

2 tablespoons (16 g) carob powder

3 tablespoons (27 g) coconut sugar

1. In a small saucepan over low heat, warm the coconut milk for 2 to 3 minutes.

2. Whisk in the coconut cream until melted.

3. Whisk in the carob powder and coconut sugar until well combined. Serve warm with additional coconut cream, if desired.

RESOURCES

Anthony's Goods
coconut flour,
arrowroot starch, and
tapioca starch
www.anthonysgoods.com

Thrive Market
coconut flour, coconut
milk, arrowroot starch,
tapioca starch, and
more pantry staples.
www.thrivemarket.com

Grain Brain Organics
palm shortening
www.amazon.com

Tropical Traditions
coconut flour
www.healthytraditions.com

If You Care
unbleached
parchment paper
www.ifyoucare.com

Vitamix
high-speed blenders
www.vitamix.com

Organic Gemini
tigernut flour
www.organicgemini.com

Vital Proteins
collagen
www.vitalproteins.com

ACKNOWLEDGMENT

TO MY LOVING HUSBAND, Daniel, this book and, really, none of Unbound Wellness would exist without you cheering me on. Thank you for believing in me, for inspiring me, and for putting up with the endless parade of packages of kitchen props and vintage dresses during the months I was writing this book! I love you so much.

To the team at Fair Winds Press, thank you for all your help and hard work to make this book a reality.

To my fellow AIP bloggers, thank you for your support and for all you do to spread this important message of real food. To Dr. Sarah Ballantyne, thank you so much for all of the amazing work you do and for writing the foreword for this book.

To my family, thank you for helping me test so many recipes in this book, and for all your support. When I say, "family" that also includes Stinky the cat who posed for a photo for this book, and kept me company for the entirety of writing it.To my friend Melanie Shafranek, I couldn't imagine having anyone else but you help me with the chapter cover photography for this book. Thank you for helping bring my vision to life and sharing your talents.

To my readers, I can't even begin to describe how grateful I am for your support. Thank you for trying my recipes, for sharing your kind words, and for helping make this book a reality by encouraging me to write it!

And, above all, none of this would be possible without strength and guidance from God.

ABOUT THE AUTHOR

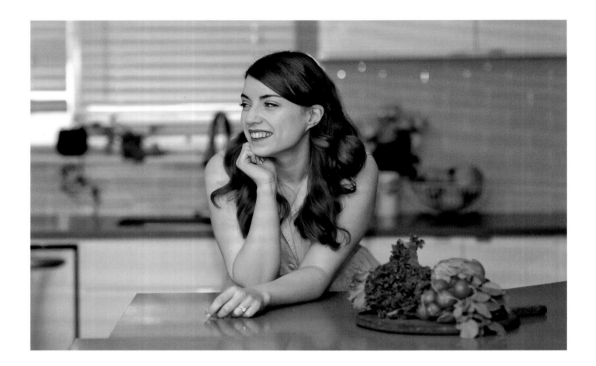

MICHELLE HOOVER was diagnosed with Hashimoto's, an autoimmune disease of the thyroid, at age 17. In an attempt to alleviate her debilitating symptoms, she began exploring a healing diet and lifestyle. However, the prospect of giving up grains, dairy, and all processed foods was daunting. Today, she specializes in making delicious healing foods that adults and kids alike will love! Michelle currently resides in Dallas, Texas, with her husband, Daniel, and their cat and spends her days running the popular recipe and health blog, UnboundWellness.com. You can find more from her on her blog and Instagram at @Unboundwellness.

INDEX